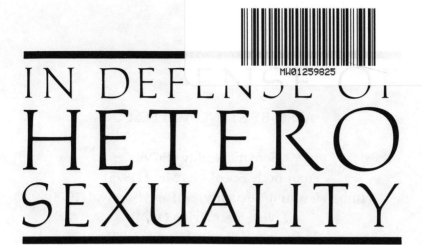

IN DEFENSE OF HETERO SEXUALITY

ALSO BY STANLEY KELEMAN

Somatic Reality (1979)
Your Body Speaks Its Mind (1975)
Human Ground/Sexuality, Self and Survival (1975)
Living Your Dying (1974)
Todtmoos: A Book of Poems (1971)

IN DEFENSE OF
HETERO
SEXUALITY

Stanley Keleman

CENTER PRESS   BERKELEY CALIFORNIA

© 1982 by Stanley Keleman
All Rights Reserved
including the right of reproduction
in whole or in part in any form

Published by Center Press
2045 Francisco Street
Berkeley, California 94709

Typesetting by Accent & Alphabet
Berkeley, California

Library of Congress Catalog Card Number: 82-83644
ISBN 0-934320-06-3

In Chapter 9 a selection is reprinted by permission of Sierra Club Books
from *The Unsettling of America* by Wendell Berry, copyright © 1977 by
Wendell Berry.

For Gail, who understands that this book
is a drama of our inner life
as well as a social viewpoint.

And for those who understand that anatomy
means the dynamic structure of experience
and is not to be confused with pictures in a book.

Contents

Acknowledgements

There are many people to thank: Gene Hendrix for his constant readiness to help with research tasks and with typing and retyping manuscripts. And Ian Grand who supported the idea for this book and who reviewed the original manuscript.

I thank my wife, Gail, for her suggestions and help, and Marilyn Brawman Haller who acted as editor and worked hours with me to bring these pages into final form.

Author's Note

Does heterosexuality need a defense? And, if so, why? Something happened a few years ago that made me realize how far we as a culture have moved. When California made requirements for its mental health workers to take special courses in human sexuality, my mail was flooded with advertisements for qualifying seminars. All these announcements taken together provided a rare overview of current thinking on sexuality. The attempt to include every possibility and give it serious academic and clinical importance made me wonder if we had reached a point where there were no longer any boundaries to sexual expression. These course offerings postulated no sexual destiny, only a psychological and social drama. Anatomy was presented as simply functional and mechanistic.

When I was asked to teach a course on sexuality for professionals, I wanted to speak out, to teach sexuality as based in biology and emotions rather than psychology and politics. I began to speak about anatomy as a living emotional process, about anatomy and feeling as the true heart of sexuality, as the fundamental basis for personal and social behavior. This book is based on these series of lectures and seminars.

Gender, the male-female bond, and even procreation itself are now being challenged. The psychological revolution begun in Vienna at the turn of the century has become part of the popular culture. We are encouraged to fantasize, to dream, to live openly the contents of our psyche, including its dark and repressed aspects.

Ever since Freud, we have been broadening the meaning of male and female and their relationship to each other. Sometimes it has been necessary to deny or twist biology in order to support certain psychological notions, such as bisexuality or androgyny. Although the free exploration of images can enhance psychic and emotional growth, we cannot alter our basic human heritage as established by anatomy. We may imagine overcoming anatomical destiny, but cannot accomplish this transcendence literally. When psychology becomes disembodied, we are left with an impersonal biology which does not fit the facts of human life.

Our educational and social institutions are increasingly built on mounting distortions of information about gender. In our pluralistic society, there is a vigorous dialogue between those who believe that the world is biologically based and those who wish to shape society according to current notions of equality and personal choice. The point to appreciate is that the dynamics between these two views underlie many of the changes in our society. We tend to confuse equality with homogeneity. We confuse psychological projections with biological facts, emotional freedom with political freedom, the public world with the private world. When we undermine gender differences, we distort the truth, and, to this extent, heterosexuality does need a defense.

In writing this book I realize I may be misunderstood and misinterpreted. What I am rejecting is present-day ideas of sex as shown and dramatized in advertising, news reporting, television and cinema, and as objectified by science. Also, sexuality is now so political that one can barely make a statement about sex and love without being labeled a sexist, religious fanatic, an anti-lifer, or other epithets.

I consider myself a somatic environmentalist whose concern is to know something about somatic and emotional sanity. I seek to protect and to nurture our basic environment—our body—and not to be victim to intellectual notions and sociological idealism. My work has to do with the living experience of people, with their cells and tissues, their emotions and psyches. I see life as a living organism with patterns of evolution and personal development. I present a process view of sexuality—biological and emotional concepts which are basic to psychotherapy, education, and human development.

My concern in this book is not with individual sexual choices, but with the references that educators, legislators, and psychotherapists are using to define the thrust of life. I refer readers interested in my ideas about individual sexual maturation and its direct application to therapy to my other books, especially *The Human Ground* and *Your Body Speaks Its Mind*.

It is not my essential point that every person should have children or family. Or that the first business of adult life is to become mothers and fathers. Not at all. However, it is everyone's concern to know that the familial bond is the backbone of human society. Emotional maturity demands of each individual a recognition and acceptance of the basic facts of existence regardless of how one may choose to live his life. Throughout history, societies have included nonreproductive options for their members, but have not confused these choices with their basic heterosexual roots.

Gender is the given of human nature. We are all endowed with gender, some weakly or poorly, others strongly or excessively, but endowed we are, and this force is the most powerful factor in our emotional orientations to our sexual identities. Social forces, traditions, and dogmas can cripple a person, bend him toward or away from his gender, but not eliminate its reality.

This is a small book; its points are few and basic. I have written it to affirm the primacy of our biological and gendered ground, a ground which has intimate connections to our personal and subjective anatomical experiences. Through these connections, we are linked to a point of reference that is at once personal and planetary, giving us a sense of belonging and a place from which to evaluate and make decisions, personally and collectively. It is one of the explicit intents of this book to encourage and restore the vitality and the passion of gender.

I have every desire to avoid reading, or appearing to read, sexual symbolism into every form and function. Yet, such is the nature of the Universal Design that the root story of the universe derives a ready symbolism from the simple story of human love and marriage. For, as we shall see, the powers that impel the eternal male and the eternal female are not petty forces germane only to man, but are the epiphany in our ordinary lives of the configuration of the primal and ultimate Cosmos.

FRANCIS J. MOTT

1 / The Essentials of Existence

SOME years ago, when I began to seek an image of mankind upon which to base my own life, I pursued the ideas of various disciplines that attempted to answer the question of man's place in the universe. Psychology seemed to offer a hope for understanding the *élan vital,* and also an ideal of who man could be. But I found purely psychological descriptions of human activity to be ultimately unsatisfying, because they did not take into account the body, the soul, or a larger destiny.

Having been trained in both the healing sciences and athletics, I was attracted to approaches that tried to understand the body as the basis of existence and satisfaction. An early notion I held, using the language of the time, was "a healthy mind in a healthy body." Psychology had tried to say it the other way around: "a healthy mind makes a healthy body." But the notion of a healthy body as it was generally used was limited because it left out the idea of the person. In the popular conception, the mind dominated the body or the body dominated the mind. The attempts to reduce man to a materialistic event or to explain

2 / The Essentials of Existence

the body through metaphysical and idealistic notions were unacceptable to me. We are, I thought, more than a collection of particles in a pattern, and certainly more than the organization of impersonal energy fields or materializing entities infusing matter with life.

This dissatisfaction eventually led me to grasp that experience itself would lead me to the conception I needed. Just as Einstein was required to reject the language of Newton, I decided that we must reject both the mechanistic and the spiritualistic languages concerning the body and develop instead a vision from the actual experience of living.

I experienced myself as a connected series of events that had a unity. I thought, I dreamed, I felt, I got excited, I moved, I had concrete experiences and invisible ones. I had a hormonal existence, a muscular existence, a social existence. We have more than one body. When we go to sleep we become the body of the dreamer. When we go to work we become the body of the worker. In loving we become the body of the lover. We are at the same time one body and many bodies. My life was composed of a multiplicity of excitatory experiences in which I formed myself.

This led me to the idea of the formative process. I realized that in my experiencing I was continually organizing myself bodily, creating the shape and form of my life. This is the mystery of making a body. We are the development of a series of life shapes from childhood to adulthood, changing structures and qualities of experience. These changes are seen embryologically—a series of bodies, connecting to each other, generating other bodies. Body-making generates more body-making, experiencing generates more experiencing. We are constantly changing the shape of our structure; our experience shapes our form.

Biological process, seen outwardly, is the development of the different bodies we have in our lifetime. Experienced inwardly, it is the different realms of our subjective life. It is the process by which we organize ourselves, shape ourselves, and seek satisfaction. It is manifested as all the events and experiences that make up our lives.

The idea of biological process — somatic forming — eliminates the concept that splits experience into two realms; it allows us to see how persons form their world by their life activity, gestures, imagery, and feeling. This conception helped me to understand the formative process, and this understanding led to a practical methodology of working with people. When I work with someone emotionally, I want to know what is forming somatically, what kind of person is taking shape. I want to know what the person is trying to satisfy, how desire seeks satisfaction, how feeling becomes action or thought.

In the course of this work I recognized that the human being has a given, immutable nature and at the same time is capable of many reorganizations. Life is situational. We live in a sea of constantly altering situations, in a stream of constantly changing internal and external realities, new desires, new people, new environmental conditions. A person who is capable of experiencing his process is capable of being in these changing situations in a way that is not stereotyped.

Such an individual can experience the situation he

is in rather than an image he carries with him from the past. More importantly, he is able to shape both himself and the situation, to make his world. He has a chance to modify behavior that is obsolete for his survival and to reformulate the nature of his actions and images based upon experiences. This leads to increased possibilities for physical, emotional, and intellectual satisfaction.

It is from this vision that I continue to develop a language and a work that encourages the growth of this kind of individual, a language and work that addresses the shaping of experience, and speaks of both our biological heritage and the somatic nature of daily living.

The goal of my work is to assist people in recognizing and developing an identity that comes from their own excitement and emotionality, their living process. Most people are totally identified with their social personality, their mental imagery. They are identified with the part of themselves that judges and controls their excitement, that strives to attain socially acceptable images they have introjected.

I teach people to experience themselves physically and emotionally, to feel their life choices as a pattern of bodily shaping that permits certain kinds of excitation and prohibits others. They learn to recognize the vividness of gender and to enact desire and longing, whether for food, intimacy, sex, or self-expression. When I say "bodily" I don't mean to reduce the person to the materialistic, mechanistic body implied by contemporary science. Neither do I imply an occult vaporization. I mean the concrete experience of one's existence, beginning on the ground floor of the instinctual life, where there is no separation between biology and personality.

At the heart of my concern is the cultivation of the ancient biological soup from which the currents of creation emerge. Excitement is a cosmological event, the fuel for the sun as well as for cellular activity. The generation of excitation, the transmission of energy, on a cosmological or biological level, is the basis of existence. We can talk about it as the evolution of particles, the process of photosynthesis, or as cellular replication. Each of us can experience this as a primordial, nonverbal, excitatory process that gives rise to the tides of gender, feeling, desire, imagination, and actions, moving toward the world and away, expanding and congealing itself.

The excitatory process is something we have in common, yet it is individual from person to person. Each person's excitation organizes differently, creating unique qualities by the ways it shapes itself. This notion is basic: there is an excitatory pattern. Out of the currents of liquid, hormonal flows, each person is formed as a unique male or female.

Our excitatory process teaches us directly how to generate behavior that moves toward satisfaction, or how to inhibit the movement of our excitation. We experience in our bodies both how to create various qualities and the possibility of alternate excitatory patterns. In the course of this work the source of a person's knowledge of himself changes. One learns to no longer identify with the memory of what others have told him about himself, or their analysis of his behavior. Instead the ability to recognize one's own pattern of sensation and feeling becomes the self-reference, to identify with a chain of somatic movements and events. The source of human knowing, then, is not in memory or in analytical powers, but in our biological roots. The social personality which grows out of the somatic process begins to recognize that its nourishment comes from excitation and its fulfillment.

Gender is at the foundation of our individual beings and heterosexuality is the basis upon which human society is built. There is a trend to turn away from these essential, enduring, biological and emotional truths, and to construct rules and values based upon the ideals of personal freedom and self-enhancement. Such shifts in standards have consequences that are at once obvious and elusive, some of which can be observed in the confused sexual values that have entered our culture. Sex roles and family structure are changing, as the primary interest of many men and women is to realize themselves as individuals and to work for high income and professional goals, rather than to work for the family.

What concerns me is that in the quest for individual freedom, heterosexuality is depreciated and loses its thrust and its potential for sustaining humanness. This book has not been written either to support or deny marriage, monogamy, or the choices of the ascetic or homosexual. It is written to affirm heterosexuality as the ground floor of human life, and to show the varying levels and meanings of a gendered existence.

Sexual truths are increasingly obscured behind physiological and statistical data. Such scholarly pornography contributes to an ethos in which some of the simplest facts about the functions of mating and reproduction are neglected or demeaned. William J. Bennett, writing in the *American Educator*, describes the ethos that is formed by the attitudes, precepts, and actions of adults. When adults behave and talk about sex in ways that support the isolation of sexual activity, it becomes a thing divorced from the emotional bonds and passions between men and women. This ethos, then, becomes the social context in which individual sexual activity takes place.

Sex is treated as a recreation, an itch to be scratched, as some sexual researchers would have it. The message coming from the middle-class adult world is caution and precaution but not restraint. In this cultural ethos, sexual activity is permitted, but the "consequences" of sexuality are to be avoided. Sex in any form, at any time, but never for procreation. Don't get pregnant and don't contract "social" diseases.

Therapists and counselors too often support these notions by encouraging uncommitted sexuality and sex for easy gratification, discounting by omission its seriousness and mystery. Little or nothing is said about the value of restraint and maturity, or of the power inherent in the emotional nature of sexuality, or the struggles that are part and parcel of heterosexual bonding. The values of family and long-term relationship are considered too parochial, restrictive, or boring. The dramatic increase in single-parent families is testimony to this modern version of freedom. Not only are there fewer and fewer models for successful heterosexual bonding, but we, as a culture, are moving farther away from the enduring truths that heterosexual interaction has to teach.

How could this alienation have come about? I think of it as the Harlow syndrome. Harry Harlow, the animal researcher, showed that monkeys, separated from their mothers, grew up with serious problems socially and sexually. They became violent and sexually confused about their roles; if impregnated, the females had hostile, destructive, murderous rages toward their offspring. It seems to me that our present cultural confusion about the functions and the evolution of heterosexuality is producing similar results. A new generation of people is complaining about isolation and alienation, and a loss of social satisfaction.

When we disturb the procreative instincts and distort the meaning of gender, we diminish some of the deepest emotions and most selfless aspirations of which mankind is capable: the nurturing and love of children and the building of a more humane world for coming generations. This book, in part, is a reminder about the obvious facts of human existence. There are foundational, evolutionary truths about heterosexual behavior. Male and female are distinct and different qualities, participating together within a reproductive intelligence — a replicating heterosexual logic that is expressed in the roles of mating and nesting and nurturing offspring. This heterosexual intelligence has brought us to where we are today, and it continues to make the future possible. Its concerns are different from a non-reproductive logic that supports primarily the enhancement of personal freedom with no real concern for future generations.

"Anatomy is destiny," Freud said in 1912. That means our bodies are our fate. When we are born in a man's or a woman's form, we are destined to have certain experiences. This is a powerful truth that took me a long time to appreciate. Over the years, I have come to respect the determining force of our biological nature—qualities inherent in tissues and organs. The quality of tissue tonus, healthy or weak, combined with organ motility (the pattern of movement of heart, genitals, and visceral tubes) has an intensity and a rhythm. The rhythms give rise to emotions and directly influence maleness and femaleness. A strong heart, for example, beating through the full scope of its expansion and contraction, certainly gives rise to a sense of self-confidence, vigor, and vitality. The uterus can send waves of longing for impregnation and children through a woman's body.

The sensations arising from male or female hormones and organs give an internal experience of gender and are the basis of self-knowledge, behavior, and roles in the world. Gender has survival value in an evolutionary process that begins with impersonal sexual behavior and, stage by stage, forms a personal relationship of caring and commitment that leads to individuation.

Biology is our destiny, but our bodies are not fixed, finite, mechanical machines. Rather, our bodies are a process, a living chain of events. Some events are biochemical, some are emotional and psychological, some cognitive, and some social. We exist over time in many shapes: infant, child, adolescent, adult. We exist as reproductive bodies, fathers and mothers, as well as working and creative structures. Although psychological denial of maleness or femaleness is possible, we cannot deny or hide gender physically.

Our bodies are never impersonal; they are male or female.

On the most basic biological level, it is the responsibility of the male to generate and transmit his seed, just as it is the responsibility of the female to receive this seed and give birth. This does not mean that every man and woman must literally reproduce. But this implicit intelligence of the gendered structure is built in, like breathing, an unconscious activity. Human consciousness can alter the program in an individual, but not in the race. This imperative is never the lesser part of our biological intelligence.

The use of contraception to interrupt reproduction has contributed to an infatuation with a personal state of pleasure and excitement. Individual narcissism has grown to such an extent that the basic rules of existence have been confused. Current sexual politics have further contributed to the denial or distortion of basic truths. Some would have us believe that social forces determine everything. But how could gender and procreative roles be socially determined? Mating occurs in a programmed way through the entire animal kingdom, and we are human animals. Is the human cortex alone responsible for all evolution and all disease? Do we believe that there is no destiny larger than man's?

The essentials of existence, including heterosexuality, comprise a destiny that transcends individual choice. Yet man is capable of learning different ways to enact biological rules. We learn to live our individual truth within the boundaries and demands of community. Between the polarities of raw instinct and social conformity we have a third choice—the personal sphere. This choice makes possible the development of a personal life based upon the imperative of desire. Human sexual emotions are very closely related to genetic biochemistry. After all, sexual arousal is meant to insure reproduction through mating. Desire, interest, variety, are part of the dynamic between men and women. Sexual arousal and role behavior are deeply linked reproductively. They are always together in a social relationship, although they are not necessarily congruent, just as arousal and object choice are not always linked.

Males and females do not always choose their opposites. Homosexual love, though free from the forces of procreation, is not free from the roles rooted in anatomy. Homosexual partners live out a version of male and female, a further indication of the inborn nature of gender and gendered roles. Homosexuality is an orientation that, in some instances, is destined and, in others, a result of personal experience and social upbringing. Nonetheless, heterosexuality reflects an imperative of nature that is destined for most of humanity.

There is a place for alternate sexual choices and, at the same time, there are parameters to human existence that are given, that influence behavior. These parameters mix with social forces, which are powerful in their own right, and play an enormous role in influencing the way we act out our roles and the choices we make.

While there are many choices, there is only one reproductive life I know about. While there are many ways to raise children, I only know of one sure way to

conceive and birth them. I am not for denying anyone's choice, but I am against creating confusion,
especially in the young and immature, who have
limited experience from which to understand human
nature. Our society needs only to be secure in its
biological heritage without confusion; it need not
deny anyone's personal liberty or choice.

Especially, one sees confusion between procreative roles and simple division of labor, and between
sex and love. Sex as recreation or entertainment is
mistaken for emotional intimacy. Sexual love and the
freedom to choose the object of one's desire are now
considered as a goal for maturity, rather than the
intimacy that comes with long-term relationship. The
psychiatrist and author M. Scott Peck has written that
the notion of love as a simple, effortless, welling-up
of passion is a destructive myth because it leaves
people unprepared for life's most important stresses.
It suggests that what is arduous is defective, and that
gratifications deferred are gratifications unattainable.
The ability to defer gratification is an attribute of
maturity. "Love," says Peck, "is always either work
or courage."

Our society also confuses the symbolic and the
concrete. Bisexuality, or the androgyne, is an example. Both sexes have within themselves male and
female hormones and both have nurturing and fe-
cundating functions. Both have potential for assertion and receptivity, passion and tenderness. The
ideal of a complete and whole nature does not mean
that men should be women or should act as women
sexually, or vice versa; such notions confuse the truth
of anatomical destiny, the symbolic with the real. As

Joseph Campbell, the American mythologist and scholar, has often pointed out, some of human history's most desperate chapters have occurred when symbols and myth have been acted upon literally.

It would be less than the whole truth to say that gender and reproductive roles are an interaction between nurture and nature. Reproductive sexual roles are more than inclinations; they are innate. What can be learned and adapted are the ways to live out these roles. After all, what would the fate of mankind be if the reproductive roles were eliminated? The consequences are almost impossible to imagine.

Sexuality and sexual roles, then, include both the given and the learned. We can learn to fuse tenderness and assertion, to extend and nurture the emotional bonds that provide the ground for intimacy and satisfaction. What we can learn is a broader view. For a moderate number of people, reproductive denial is possible for a time; for some, it is possible for a lifetime. But for the majority, the reproductive drama, family bonding, and participation in a future cannot be denied. The roots of humanity lie in the heterosexual imperative.

2 / Sexuality as Emotional Process

OVER the last twenty-five years there has been a fundamental reappraisal of the nature of human sexuality. The questions concern such provocative issues as what sexual performance is all about, what orgasm is, what is permissible and what is taboo, what is natural and what is not, what is the nature of male and female identity, and what is the place of family and child rearing in our society. Such questioning has led to an out-pouring of opinions and experimentation at all levels of the society, which in turn has given rise to a flood of authorities claiming to deal with the fundamental issues of sexuality. Yet there are few texts that speak of the essential somatic nature of sexuality: the destiny of anatomy linked with the emotion of our humanness — the union of sex and love.

Human sexuality is a biological, psychological, and emotional process, a chain of somatic events that give shape and meaning to the continuum of our personal lives. It is emotional involvement that transforms an impersonal biological process into a human one — into an act of love.

Human sexual satisfaction depends upon the givens of biology and the history of emotional arousal. The peaks and valleys of the hormonal tides and the sensations of anatomy are important, but not more important than the interactions that make up our emotional history. Together these set the tone for psychological and sexual dispositions.

Sexual nature begins in the womb with the connection to our mother's body. We are either wanted or not, enjoyed and cared for or not. This is the feeling connection that begins to give our emotions a future. After birth, a child is fed with love and caring or indifference and dislike. The brain grows and the heart is committed to the nature of the responses we receive as baby girls and boys. At puberty, the body changes again, becoming more specifically male or female; the brain is flooded with hormones and the responses of our parents and peers to our sexuality. We either get or do not get the support to be ourselves and live a gendered and emotional life. The early feelings of connection, the bonding with mother and family, form the emotional history that connects us with our personal past, supports us in the present, and leads us to the future. These feelings are the basis of self-love and love shared with others.

Sexual satisfaction requires emotional and visceral experience. Our sexual process is how we live the quantities and qualities of excitation and feeling; how our organ motility permits and encourages the forming of feelings — those passionate and powerful experiences within ourselves and between people. The way we learn emotionally is our destiny. When we learn to use ourselves with affection and assertion, we learn to relate to others with care and strength. Caring and affection, though, are not all there is to the emotional base of sexuality. There is power — the feelings of passion and intensity, domination and acceptance, self-interest and satisfaction.

The ongoing drama of heterosexuality is in the experiences and feelings that arise from our anatomy and form into patterns of intimacy and individuality. Heterosexuality involves directly the feeling process of building deep and powerful sexual bonds that facilitate emotional and psychological maturity.

Sexuality, then, is linked with emotions because it is an outgrowth of personal history as well as anatomy. The development of our somatic feelings deeply affects sexual identity and lovemaking styles. In sexual activity, you enter the instinctual world as well as the social world. But if you are unmotivated by your gender, or if you lack the ability to share your private experience, to mingle your emotions and to be affected by your passions, if you are unable to transmit caring and passion, tenderness and intensity, you are less than you can be.

The multiplicity of lifestyles that are available today due to the acceptance of contraception is a great blessing. The person who wishes to be non-reproductive, and yet sexual, can live a happy life, unplagued by religious or social stigmas. We have become free to express ourselves, to be more of ourselves. This freedom has a tragic and dangerous side, however. And this is in undermining some of the truths that heterosexuality and the reproductive life teach. Male and female are different in ways that are deep and enduring and are the basis for reproduction and family, for long-term bonding and the perpetuation of love. Human sexuality evokes emotional life, forming ties of intimacy and individuality.

In recent years, there has been an attack, both subtle and blatant, on the feelings and roles of male and female and on the place of family and commitment. Many people in our culture want to emphasize similarities, and not differences. Sex is equated with instant gratification and fantasy. There is professional literature on sexuality that explains sex as a mechanical function, no more than stimulus-response. It is as if human sexuality functioned like a machine, to be wired to perform this way or that. Too many current approaches to sexuality deliberately and continually divorce it from the emotional development of the individual. There is a concentration on technique and performance, on descriptions of sexuality as mechanical programs, orgasmic catharsis, or narcissistic fulfillment.

When the media promote the idea that certain appearances and behavior make a person desirable, sex becomes a fantasy divorced from our deepest urges. Sex becomes disembodied and exploitive. Our population is bombarded by ideas, pictures, and dramas sensationalizing sex and linking it with fear, hostility, and murder. The main source of arousal becomes fantasies related to adrenalized feelings. Sex equals shoot and kill. Men are portrayed as steely, macho warriors or sleek, feminine boys; women as exaggerated amazons or mannish girls. Impersonal, stereotyped appearances and behavior become the goal. There is nothing in these approaches that speaks either of the intimacy of our somatic rhythms or of the emotional bonding that creates personal individuality and the communion with others that most people hunger for today. Sexual intimacy has more to offer than the storms of excitatory ecstasy and the indulgence of catharsis that many people think they want. It is more than a spontaneity that is really mindlessness. What real sexual satisfaction has to offer is the forming of a life that is connected to the basic elements of existence, not only sexual union, but the thrust of being a passionate, emotionally alive person.

What is essential to my view is that sexuality is part of a bigger process. It doesn't stand by itself. Human sexuality is a multi-layered emotional experience. Its ground is the very essence of being — from the mystery of creation and desire to forming a union where the thrust of our caring transcends self-interest by creating blood connections with others. Sexuality is the continuation of our personal histories of being cared for, giving us many layers of subjective meaning and value that provide a whole range of satisfactions.

Our innate organ motility, our inner hormonal tides, and our emotional connection with others extend the excitatory process into feelings called love. It is this socialized excitement that signifies the difference between emotionally based sexuality and techniques of behavior engineering, which have little to do with helping a person learn how to live passionately or how to continue the deep arousal patterns of love. It is the experience of deeply satisfying visceral motility connected to psychological and interpersonal responses that is important. This emotional layer makes sexuality a living, human process, rather than a mechanical or programmed appetite to be slaked.

Our sexual process is an emotional wave that gives us continuity, that anchors us in our past and helps us avoid its pains while in the present we seek satisfaction. This is the key and the clue to the nature of heterosexuality — that it is an emotional reality.

3 / The Three Realms

LIFE can be said to have three layers, or realms, like a cell. The first layer is in contact with the outer world, where its shape is always changing; the central layer, the nucleus, is where the secrets of reproduction and protein building are; the middle layer is where the actions of immediate need are dealt with. I call these the *postpersonal*, the outer ring, or societal way; the *prepersonal*, the inner ring, or nature's way; and the *personal*, the middle ring, or our way. They express the ways in which experience and function can be understood. The prepersonal is the realm of the primordial organismic function. It is here that chromosomal and anatomical sexual differentiation come into being, and here that primary arousal patterns develop for contact and closeness. The postpersonal is the realm of societal experience, where we learn what behavior and roles we are expected to embody in the conduct of our sexuality. The personal realm is the growth of individuality, the formation of our own patterns of sexuality, and the development of loving and intimacy in our personalities.

In humans the prepersonal realm is the realm of

the impersonal, prior to societal tradition and the development of personality, a realm of hormonal floods and primitive urges toward mating and replicating. The prepersonal world can be equated with noncortical functioning or with intrauterine life. At this level, the organism does not have an elaborate and sophisticated cortex with which to organize experience. The behavior patterns are more or less undifferentiated and highly ritualized, and are lived unselfconsciously. In the prepersonal world, the organism and the world are one. There is no self-reflection, and the individual is immersed in the environment, with little or no subjective experience of his own. The prepersonal state is like dream or myth, where creation and death are linked. It is where sex is a blind urge, where feeding and copulation go together. Here sex is short lived; intercourse is brief, and the sole purpose is union of sperm and egg. Images in the literature of natural, spontaneous sexuality come from this prepersonal realm. Typical descriptions of this kind of functioning are "it's pure sex," "the body takes over," "it's mindless," "spontaneous."

In the prepersonal world, sexuality is unrestrained nature. It is an awesome experience to find oneself experiencing the depths of this layer and to become part of the impersonality of the reproductive urges. Many mature people who are able to experience a broad range of possibilities return to these places of cosmic union, mingling again in the archetypal waters of subcortical images where destiny reigns.

The postpersonal realm is represented by society, and it has a tremendous impact upon the individual in its demand for compliance and strict role performance. All societies institutionalize reproductive, sexual, and courtship behavior. Sexual rules are linked directly with creation and reproduction, and certain sexual behavior and roles are obligatory. The more rigid a society, the more strict its regulation of sexual behavior. For example, sexual behavior is not permissible until a certain age; women should be virgins at the time of marriage, men need not; sex is not permitted outside of marriage. The function of such rules is to manage sex for control of reproduction and child rearing. They provide guidelines in deciding who is responsible for the offspring of sexual unions and how these children are to be raised, the division of labor, and the roles to be played. Some regulations are more liberal than others. However, even the exceptions to the rules, such as diversions from monogamy, are well ritualized and well ordered. In every culture, breaking sexual taboos has clear penalties, such as flogging, branding, ostracism, and economic deprivations.

Today social pressure to imitate public images is enormous. The proliferation of images in the public media, and even in the professional literature, too often puts us at the mercy of what we think society expects of us. Rather than learn from experience over time, we try to imitate instant images. When we are not encouraged to develop experiential references, but instead try to guide ourselves through images only, the emotional personality is underdeveloped. There is a confused avoidance of personal choice for the sake of a generalized, impersonal model. For example, women are told that there is something wrong if they don't achieve orgasm. The goal of orgasm replaces a whole range of movements and personal experiences that lead toward satisfaction. The private world is intruded upon by public pressure for performance. There is a kind of exhibitionism that pervades our lives, leaving no room for mystery or privacy.

Furthermore, we have a situation where the societal postpersonal realm is infused with prepersonal and non-human images. Previously culture tended to denigrate the prepersonal world and its animal images. ("Don't behave like a beast!") Today the raw animal is the ideal. The prepersonal responses have been transferred to the domain of the postpersonal. Here the ideal is to be able to surrender to the non-human, be it the impersonal forces of nature or the forces of the disembodied spirit. Evil has entered the sexual world with images of bondage and masochism; we hear of sex with animals, group sex where people use sex as an attack, and, lately, sexual reproduction without a mate. Sex has become a notion, a thing to do to get a sensation. We have learned to believe that images are feelings, and are stunned to discover the difference between feeling and fantasy.

People are confused by the failure of our institutions to support family, emotional maturity, and love. We are living in the aftermath of an LSD ethic, an unbounded psycho-political distortion of current psychological findings, where everything goes. The culture presents us with images of men and women as sex objects, of adultery, sexual violence, and child pornography — images from a prepersonal state. There is public encouragement to seek satisfaction for past instinctual deprivations; to seek sexual equality instead of accepting sexual differentiation; to demand instant gratification and underplay loyalty, commitment, and struggle. The model is a mythic garden of hedonistic leisure, where men and women demand all their political and biological rights as adults without having to work for them or develop the skills to create lasting relationships, emotional bonding, or family. Is it any wonder that people are confused about their sexuality, their roles, and their gender?

Many people are trapped in the dialectic between prepersonal instinct and postpersonal societal demands. They live out their lives and never develop a personal life. In the prepersonal world, the urge to fornicate lives us. We are driven and compelled by nature. In the postpersonal world, society lives us, demanding that we conform to its images by acting out the dictums of the current crop of authorities. Most people are concerned with the relationship between performance and pleasure, and organize their interpersonal communication around public expectations of what sex is supposed to be and what they should feel. They judge themselves in accordance with support or rejection from the public domain. Sexuality becomes performance dependent upon societal and familial rules, not personal choice.

In the prepersonal world we are aroused by forces beyond ourselves. We are made sexual by the programs of hormonal, genetic appetites. These patterns of innate arousal give rise to attraction and a sense of identity. Here we experience the feel of raw power and domination, of submission and reception. The ways in which we translate these basic life urges are how we develop a personal existence. In the personal realm, we learn to perpetuate or curtail the pull of desire and to coordinate muscle and visceral motility with the brain to produce social expressions of assertion and tenderness. The sustainment of feeling and expression gives rise to the images, the meanings, and the values that give sex its intimacy, its private structure, its psychological and emotional impact, and makes the personal world the human arena.

The erosion of sexuality in the modern age has occurred because the institutions that dictate sexual mores have moved from one extreme to the other — from the postpersonal and its stereotypes to the prepersonal realm where the body has been made the captive of cathartic, orgiastic rituals. The initiatory behavior of sex and love is turned into a public event, producing emotionally jaded and sexually satiated people.

In the personal realm lies the unique human function, the way of experiencing we recognize as our own. The personal realm functions in terms of experience, feeling, and cognition rather than the more easily marketable stimulation of the senses and idealization of fantasies. Societal pressure to be supernatural, super-spontaneous, and super-hedonistic produces more prepersonal orientation and less personal and social orientation, diminishing individual human satisfactions.

Personal sex is the ability to make emotional choices that modify the reproductive imperative and convert it into the multiple, but particular, ways that lead to satisfaction. Personal sex allows the prepersonal and postpersonal realms to be mediated by the richness of our personal childhood experiences. To make the impersonal personal is to nurture and make tender the dominion of love, to make the world a bit more secure. If prepersonal sexuality is a storm of programmed urges, personal sex gives raw arousal its meaning and makes of the storm an intimate, private pool of widening satisfaction. Prepersonal sexuality involves excitatory intensity, a sense of destiny, and the dominating rhythms of hunger and rest. But such waves of desire have to be translated so that pelvic and visceral motility can be coordinated into expressions of assertion and of tenderness that reflect our own and our partner's needs.

Sexuality is a continuum that starts *in utero* and progresses through infancy, childhood, adolescence, and adulthood into our elderly years. The herald of sexual, social, and personal gender preferences is at the chromosomal level, where the cellular organization is already galvanized into male or female. Concomitantly there is anatomical differentiation with the growth of sexual ducts and the specialized organs of the uterus and gonads. This internal development is followed by further specialization, and hormonal and morphological development that deepens gender. The internal growth is followed by the forming of external organs: penis, scrotum, vagina, and, later, breasts and hair. When the child enters the world, observation of the genitalia dictates society's responses to what is there: "It's a boy" or "It's a girl." These responses reinforce or deny the hormonal and morphological configuration. This is a way of saying that there is societal support for what is supposed to be. This is our public body.

The child is expected to learn to delay certain impulses, hold feelings in check, and wait for gratification. During the dependency period of childhood, a child learns to inhibit himself. This begins the birth of roles, laying the ground for what a boy or girl, man or woman is supposed to act like. All of this is internalized and brought with us into adult sexuality. The way this occurs is of primary importance. The behavior and roles set for the child by his parents is postpersonal training and can be rigidly authoritarian or very lax. In either extreme, there needs to be sufficient emotional responsiveness and encouragement to permit the development of the personal realm.

Psychological research clearly demonstrates that an intimate, constant, non-threatening environment with an adequate amount of touching and caring sets the stage for a personal dimension that stands between the two worlds of the prepersonal and the postpersonal. This type of caring, continued well into the adolescent years, softens and supports prepersonal and postpersonal dogmas and allows for the possibility of a private, individual existence. Emotional and anatomical maturity is formed by the nature of our connections to others, the kinds of bonds we have made, and how we have learned to deal with misunderstandings, disappointments, and hurts. In short, it is developed through experimental behavior, role practice, social rehearsal, and body posturing.

Our personhood finds strength through practice and mastery of the use of ourselves, the discovery of our own meaning, and acting upon that meaning. This all grows out of a particular way of being alive. When images and feelings about ourselves and others are organized as individuated gestures instead of programmed ones, we have learned the secret of forming a personal pattern.

This learning continues throughout our lives. We are constantly aroused and capable of new responses. This process or responsiveness can be extended over time. Repeating an action has the effect of prolonging or curtailing arousal. Images, feelings, and actions from the prepersonal world are used by tradition and ritual to increase sexual duration, just as our way of using our experience personally extends arousal. We continually move back and forth between the three realms of functioning. In the same way, the development of human sexuality leads to the development of long-term arousal patterns, which distinguishes it from the sexuality of other animals. Humans bring their unique experiences to sex, making it violent and mechanical or tender and caring.

There are three kinds of intercourse in which humans can engage. The first is the brief, intense arousal of the prepersonal realm. The second is characterized by the learned performances of the post-personal realm. The third is the long rhythm of the personal realm, where there is a harmony among the self, the other person, and their combined histories. From this rhythm we can affirm and create a richer personal life.

Prepersonal love lasts as long as one's self interest; societal love lasts as long as social interest demands. The long rhythm in sex is developed in the family, when the brain begins to support the somatic history of its own experience, to take the short-term patterns and extend them.

Without the involvement of the personal realm,

sex is a compulsion that insures survival and only transitory pleasure. Emotional development is not guaranteed, only relief. In the personal realm, we use the rhythms that connect us to the prepersonal and the postpersonal. In prepersonal sexuality, there is impulsiveness, a wild rush to enter, to submit, to be mindless, to be at one with the gushes of desire. In postpersonal sexuality there are concepts like the good boy, the good girl, gentleman, hero, virgin, wife, mother, husband, and father. In the personal world there is the choice of romantic love and growth of maturity that promises enduring friendship and intimacy. Here one can contain the intensities of excitement, the sense of the self, and the ability to enact needs — to be societal or instinctual or both.

Most of us were not reared in what could be called ideal family situations, with the result that there will be aspects of sexual functioning that have not been allowed to develop and mature. Some adults, for example, are fixed at a stage in their prepersonal development in which sexuality is basically childlike or infantile. The partner is an object and sex is an impersonal, ritualized performance. Some adults are able to invoke only short-term patterns of prepersonal genital organization, and are incapable of extended tenderness, intimacy, and caring. Others may need to repetitiously reenact the postpersonal roles. This may happen in spite of personal preferences or longings for less constrained and more satisfying roles. For others, difficulties exist in the personal realm: one can be capable of intimacy and personal presence, yet out of touch with the powerful urges of the prepersonal realm.

Sexual pleasure and intimacy, psychological and physiological satisfaction are capable of being learned and of being altered through learning. That is to say, sexual maturity is learned. The prepersonal world grows, as do the personal and postpersonal realms, each in their time. The secret is that they must be practiced in order to grow. We have the given and we have the learned. Many a person has an adult body but never engages in adult activity except with his brain. As adults we have the possibility of recognizing in ourselves what aspects of sexuality have become fixed and have not been allowed to mature, and we can then learn for ourselves the conditions that will allow us to mature.

As we identify the roles we are playing and the desires that have not been allowed to deepen to satisfaction, we have the opportunity to learn to live as fully as possible in all three realms, increasing the dimensions of our intimacy and deepening our expressions of satisfaction.

This is the heterosexual drama — the deepening of sexual intimacy, the privilege of riding the wave of the formative process that builds essential emotional bonds. Heterosexuality is like being on an escalator, riding up and down between prepersonal sexual desire, socially defined love, and personal love. It is the maturation of desire into affection and the caring for self and others that both individuates and transcends the self and represents the hope for a truly human biosphere.

4 / Arousal and Inhibition

IF we are to understand sexuality and gender, and if
we want to know what satisfaction is, we have to look
at the nature of arousal and its inhibition, since it is
here that patterns of movement and action develop.
Arousal and how it is sustained and managed is the
story of our sexual lives.

Arousal calls forth desire through the intensification of excitement and cellular motility, and it is capable of maturing into feeling and form. Through inhibition, arousal is intensified as motility is delayed.
This holding pattern allows sensations of excitement
to build up and become feeling. The slowing down of
motility allows appropriate action patterns to form.

Behavior begins as undifferentiated excitement
caused either by internal cellular motility or the
external world. For example, we are aroused by
hungers for air or for food, by our hormones and
feelings, as well as from the simple mechanical movement of our bodies in space.

Sexual arousal springs from all levels of somatic
process. Imagination is a tool of arousal; it arises from
the same primary process, anchored in our biology

and emotions. Imagination and excitement are linked, encouraging greater intensity, self-knowledge, sexual diversity, and pleasure.

Image-making is gendered; it is not neuter. Chromosomal differentiation sets the pattern of metabolism that becomes the images that then seek to evoke mating responses from its opposite. Inner sexual identity comes from chromosomal development, biochemical hormonal givens, and through the formation of anatomical organs and their position.

Our internal identity contains the ancient archetypes of maleness and femaleness, with all the feelings and sensations and associations that make us unusual and individual. Inner self images are not only pictures; they are psychological, emotional, and biochemical. These images enhance gender and maintain the excitatory continuum. Severe inhibition of the excitatory process can result in the disembodiment of the image-making function. Imagination when not connected to the biological self becomes fantasy. A person can come to have disembodied images of his own sexuality and that of others which are impersonal and inhuman. Fantasy seeks to derive pleasure from itself, not to seek responses from others.

Fantasy life cannot be confused with inner life. Inner life consists of a pattern of excitement, feeling associations and organ motility that has a specific image. Our inner world is illuminated by internal images. They serve to communicate the needs and growth patterns of an organismic thrust toward maturity. These images and pictures give a sense of life's drama and how we can alter, rehearse, enhance our inner needs and our connection to others.

Excitement, or need that comes from the depth of one's being, will find its way toward the surface of the body, where the social world is met. This internal movement is translated into patterns of action by the human brain and muscle system. These patterns form our personal rituals of social expression, which are intended to satisfy internal needs. Our desire inspires a dance that describes us.

Arousal and inhibition have a developmental history. At every stage there is a learning, a shaping of the organism to encourage or subdue the generation of desire and to shape the patterns of our movement in the world. There is a continuum of arousal that lays down the foundation of each person's particular pattern of relating to others. First, there is self-arousal; then there is the stimulation that comes from contact, with the mother and others, in tactile and verbal conversations. This personal history of arousal indicates the relationships we have had with ourselves and others. It is personalized in the way we have learned to excite and satisfy others and ourselves.

The emotional history of parenting and the patterns of caring and response in the family are the basis for individual role building, and they give arousal social possibilities. This history also forms a person's erotic nature. A child may learn to subdue his excitement and not share it. In playing the role of "good boy" or "good girl," the child may learn to hold back his anger or pleasure. As he grows older, he learns to inhibit and separate the tender and caring excitement from genital excitement.

The clue to the embodiment of arousal and inhibition is found in the nature and function of muscle. There is in all muscle a rhythmic, wave-like quality. Smooth muscle, the muscle of viscera and organs, is responsible for the movement of material, and makes sensation inside us. There are movements of peristalsis through the digestive tract, waves of expansion and contraction of the heart and blood vessels, the waves of expansion and contraction of the womb in sexual activity and childbirth, and the pulsations of the erect penis. These waves generate deep feelings and are the source of spontaneity and feelings of self.

Visceral spaces, the hollows, the centers of our tubes — whether gut, penis, or vagina — are maintained by smooth muscle. By swelling and shrinking, these muscles are able to hold things, pass them along, to incubate or assimilate, or to incorporate and expel. In hollow spaces, feeling is increased and decreased by what fills the spaces and how they are emptied. These hollow spaces, supported by the peristaltic waves of muscle motility, give a feeling of gender. The sensations coming from the uterus and vagina and the sensations coming from the penis are different. Sexual identity is strengthened by the brain's recognition of these internal sensations and movements. Internal organ motility is the basis for our deepest satisfaction and sexual identity.

For example, there are rhythmic pulsations in the mouth that are reinforced by the whole body when the digestive and breathing tubes function in a grasping, penetrating, and pulling-in manner. The same powerful rhythms are experienced in sex — the reaching of the vagina, its powerful sucking movements, and the penetrating movements of the penis. These movements act with the pelvis to make an action like a cylinder — sucking back and thrusting forward — helping to exchange the nourishment of sensations and bringing out the fluids that make fertilization possible. The intense rhythm of the hollows is the inside of ourselves speaking. When this is shared with another, we create a deep bond. The cavity of the heart has intense pulsations, as do the uterus, the penis, and the brain. Anything that interferes with this pulsation diminishes feeling from the insides, weakens sexual assertiveness and identity, and, without question, decreases our satisfaction.

Patterns of rhythmicity in muscle can be inhibited or altered. The movements of swelling and sucking are pleasurable, and to prolong that pleasurable, rhythmical pattern requires inhibition or extension. This is how the brain and skeletal muscles work together. The brain and skeletal muscles inhibit so that learning can take place. We delay the immediate responses so that new patterns can form. We inhibit crying and learn to ask for what is needed. We learn to prolong movements that give us a sense of self.

Patterns of arousal and inhibition are also patterns of learning. The excitatory configurations of rhythmical patterns evoke a multiplicity of responses from others and lead to relationships with the world. There is an innate desire for self-management, a wish to master our own excitement. This is the basis for learning sexual satisfaction. We have the ability to prolong excitement. The ability to use volition to inhibit the automatic movements gives new feeling and expression. Extending rhythmical movements allows them to develop and to become the source of satisfaction. This growth is learned, and must be practiced to ripen.

The postponing of immediate gratification or action in response to desire has served to perpetuate the clan, the tribe, and the family through the creation of tradition and ritual. The inhibition of arousal was originally intended to develop self-management and to make community possible, although it was later used to suppress prepersonal behavior and to enforce political and religious dogmas.

Brain-skeletal muscle satisfactions (learned behavior) can become confused with the profound satisfactions that emerge from the smooth muscles of organs. Personal maturity depends on the participation of both systems, the voluntary and involuntary, the coordination between feeling and action. To intensify and elongate feelings in the visceral organs and smooth muscle, to coordinate them through brain and skeletal muscle for appropriate behavior, is our challenge. The coordination of these two behaviors reaches its highest expression in personal bonding.

Social personality is built on individual ways of inhibition. The mechanism of role creation is intimately related to inhibition in the muscular and skeletal systems. Inhibition is the necessary component of synthesis and facilitation. The ability to delay is the ability to make boundaries and is the first step in generating identity. In the postpersonal or social world, self-control is demanded. The societal group functions as a teaching environment, sharing collective experiences of inhibition that lead to muscular-cognitive mastery. We learn by imitating general patterns of behavior and then making them more specific. These specific behaviors enable us to recognize who we are. Social roles become like suits of clothes; we can take them out and put them on for different occasions. Unfortunately, we sometimes identify too much with these roles and think of ourselves as defined solely by our social performances. In the past, society has demanded an extreme control of arousal. But, in recent years, we have been told the opposite; the goal is to be instantly and continuously excited, rather than to learn the behavior that facilitates the continuous development of a feeling life.

Sexuality has an intimate connection with arousal. Hormonal juices enliven the male and female anatomy, urging each toward specific roles. Societal models either facilitate or discourage the urges of nature, but social roles alone do not give a person true identity. If motility has been severely limited, then the sensations coming from the tissues create feelings of inadequacy or low libido.

The difference between social roles and tissue motility is at the root of the confusion between what does and does not lead to satisfaction. The muscles that move the pelvis forward and back serve to prolong and intensify the excitement that supports the arousal of the penis and uterus. This stimulation keeps the penis erect and opens the vagina and uterus. When the pelvic movement is too inhibited or is forced, excitement becomes shallow. If the movement is allowed to follow innate patterns of intensification, it will become a wave, an emotional swelling and shrinking. This rhythmical action of mutual pelvic rocking gives powerful contact and is our connection with the ancient biological functions and the emotions of our personal history. It is this wave of movement that touches another and bonds feeling to expression.

Many sexual difficulties can be traced to problems of arousal or inhibition. When inhibition is weak, or when there is an inability of brain or muscle to delay, then feeling and action are not coordinated in a way that leads to satisfaction. Where there is lack of arousal, excitement cannot form into action. If inhibition is too severe, there is a need for strong stimulation to overcome depression. Whichever way, when arousal and inhibition are diminished, so is intimacy.

Many people have excitement but do not allow it to ripen into intimacy. Others, who work hard at being terrific lovers and claim to have mastered the techniques of stimulation and sexual movement, often remain emotionally deprived and substitute rehearsed mechanical actions for deeper organic motility. When excitement is localized in the genitals, movements are exaggerated and limited. If tissue is not responsive, intimacy suffers. Some men, for example, try to sustain excitement by squeezing themselves. Some women become mere receptacles for the aggressive and thrusting penetration of men because this is what makes sensation for them.

Over-inhibited or under-inhibited, over-aroused or under-aroused, any of these states discourages the long-term arousal patterns which support the emotions that develop into intimacy. Mechanical, unfeeling performances bring about boredom and apathy. Mature arousal and inhibition go together as one function. Arousal, expansion, inhibition, and containment are parts of a pattern of intensification that urges feeling to form an avenue of expression. Expression frees and focuses excitement. This process of expansion and containment forms the bonds of heterosexual love.

5 / Violence in Sexuality

I HAVE suggested that sexual satisfaction depends on an ongoing resolution of the polarity of arousal and inhibition. Too much inhibition deadens the upwelling of arousal and leads away from a feeling of our basic inner motility. Arousal without inhibition discourages the formation of personality, feeling, and love.

This same polarity exists on a societal level. The security of a rigid order can be overbearing, but too little order can lead to confusion, helplessness, and senseless violence. An overly repressive system leads to suppression, defiance, insurrection, and finally to violence. Insufficient order invites a freedom to run wild, another kind of violence.

In the pursuit of freedom man has made a rather bloody history as he has sought to eliminate those imperatives that restrain action, thought, imagination, and feeling. Today, the continuing attempt to cast off Victorian notions has led, in the psychological and emotional realms, to the zealous removal of restraint after restraint, confusing inner freedom with impulsive acting out in the world.

The image of a repressive society is out of step with the truth. We are not a sexually repressive society; we are one that is overaroused and sensorily inflated. Overstimulation is our national crisis, not repression. Television, books, schools, radio, and newspapers compete for our attention, seeking access to our senses and internal lives. There is a mushrooming assault on our brains, our hormones, our bodies.

We suffer from the promise of too much potential. We believe that there are no limits; to have limits is to be repressed, and to have everything is an inalienable right. Those who cannot have, take, be it emotional satisfaction or a life. These attitudes have led to an era of increasing violence, and have become linked to creation itself — the sexual act. Sex and violence now go together like a hand and glove.

Rape, child abuse, and other violent sexual acts are on the increase. In part these are the consequences of the misguided notion that there is no need for inhibition. The proliferation of pornographic materials is part of this trend. By pornographic I mean sex that degrades self or others, sex that is meant to exploit for individual gratification. When the other is made an object, sex becomes impersonal. Once a person is transformed into a *thing,* it is easy to be violent toward, or even kill, this thing that was once a person.

Some experts say there is no pornography, only explicit sex. Further, they state that there is no link between explicit sex and violence. Rape is correctly viewed as an act of violence. A person who belittles his victims with insults and humiliating demands is involved in hurtful acts that twist and distort sex.

These violent acts cannot be characterized as purposeless and without feeling. Indeed what is sought is only thrill. The killing of a pregnant woman in the Manson slaughter was a mutilation of femininity and an attempt to rouse passion to link the tribe with the dark excitement of sex and violence.

But the problem of sexual violence is not limited to the increasingly acknowledged incidents of rape, child abuse, and pornography. There is a surfeit of images in the media that suggest excitement in danger or relief through anger and violation. We are initiated into sexuality far removed from the experience and feelings that come from our bodies. This inundation of our senses with sexual stimuli, and the cultivation of idealized expectations of performance are an assault on our sensibilities.

Public images that divorce love from sexuality, and separate sex from bonding are an act against family and against people. Bonding, tenderness, and caring have a unique ability to prevent people from abusing each other, and it is an act of violence in itself to strip sexuality of these qualities.

How, then, to explain the presence of so much violence in sex? The answer lies in the pattern of arousal. The frustration of a developing pattern of arousal potentially leads to violence. Arousal by strong and insistent stimuli while one is unable to obtain satisfaction can cause violent attacks. By seeking thrills and fantasy over tender feeling and shared experience, the door to violence is opened.

Frustration from the social inhibition of arousal happens all the time. For purposes of hygiene and toilet training, much attention is given to the genitals of infants and young children. Being touched or touching oneself as a two- or three-year-old may be acceptable, but later is discouraged or punished. As a child grows up and is aroused by members of the opposite sex, he may respond with confusion, rejection, or hostility.

Many people become hostile to their own feelings because they have been conditioned to fear them. When desire is aroused and then thwarted, when the natural tendency to reach out is punished, the result is anger. Anger and hostility become confused with sexual satisfaction. Hostility is not assertiveness; it is the result of blocking the natural growth of assertiveness. It is a social artifact. The linking of sex and violence, then, is the result of promise and disappointment.

In human sexual relations, there are balances between assertion and tenderness, but an incorrect handling of these aspects of sexuality leads to abuse and violation. There is a dance of sexuality in balancing assertiveness with tenderness. The large muscles of the back of the body that support assertion balance with the more sensual parts in the front of the body. For sexuality to be human, there must be this blend of tenderness with assertion.

In the animal kingdom, the rituals of sex are programmed so that there is no mix-up of signals. In humans, with year-round sex, there is plenty of room for mixed signals. Vulnerable parts come to face one another, and great psychological care is required to accomplish an act that is no longer for the sole purpose of transmitting seed. The possibility of hostility being introduced from remembered experiences by either partner is as great as are the instances of inhibitory and frustrating experiences.

Furthermore, there has been a weakening of the hormonal dynamic in the evolution of the human creature. There is still a part of this with us, such as smell, the menstrual and ovulation cycles, and a trace of the heat cycle of mammals. But such a dilution of what was once so directly interpreted, with given signals and given responses, has made ambiguous the proper timing of our sexual programs, and rendered rather obscure the appropriate actions of our arousal mechanisms. The dance of tenderness and assertiveness can thus become hesitant and unsure, and is liable to the injuries of frustration and wounded experience.

It is also possible that the long human dependency period, with its protraction of arousal and inhibition, further increases the likelihood of violence as a response to sexuality. If a child is dependent and in a primal learning situation until at least eighteen to twenty years of age, he is exposed to innate instability between needs and motor control for a relatively long period of time. There is more than sufficient opportunity for the experience of arousal and inhibition emerging from these factors to turn a child-parent relationship into an adult pattern of domination: love means I beat you, humiliate you, or castrate you. It is not at all uncommon for the dance of arousal to become a remembered pattern of I arouse you, I inhibit you, I humiliate you, then we make up and make love. At its most extreme, this is a cruel ritual

that is not a primary form of sexuality, but the pro-
jection of those who feel caught in a trap.

So there is some background to our current obses-
sion with violence in sex. But the conclusion drawn
by many experts that overt hostility is essential to
sexual behavior is patently absurd. Hurting oneself,
hurting another person — how ludicrous to imagine
that this is needed as a basis of sex.

The confusion is worsened by the sexual fashions
that assail us from all directions. Provocative displays
mean look and admire, but do not touch. Clothing
that accentuates the organs of sexual arousal does not
reflect the real meaning of sexual satisfaction. Indeed,
not only does it produce frustration and the attendant
unwelcome responses, but it is an act of violence
against the true functioning of anatomy. We allow
ourselves to be overstimulated, while at the same
time abiding by social demands for restraint and self-
control. Little wonder, then, that a permissive culture
witnesses within itself a drastic and escalating
increase in all manner of violence.

The brain has become today's most important
sexual organ. We are preoccupied with our senses
and our heads. Cognitive processes move us toward
increased excitement, using the rest of the body as an
object of exploitation. This is a violence few of us
think of — the violence we do to ourselves in exhaust-
ing our organs. The media do it all the time with
sensationalism. This is how sex and orgasm come to
be in our heads, not our soma and soul.

People in a permissive society may never develop
feelings, or develop only repressed feelings. Sexual
violence may then be an attempt to make contact with

one's own feelings. A person who does not have much tenderness will probably ask to be hit or to hit in order to mobilize deeper feelings. There are many people in our culture who only feel excited when they are in danger, or angry, or abused. Others are so stimulated by public sexual images that they have no hope of ever developing personal feelings. They only act out images.

Many women feel that they have to make love frequently in order to satisfy cultural dictates of what a woman should be; this is an act of violence. A man who performs sexually in order to build up his own self-esteem is doing violence to his sexual functioning. Overstimulation and overarousal do not lead to satisfaction. This is a misuse of sexual organs and a misunderstanding of the primacy of arousal and inhibition. Foreplay and titillatory arousal, previously the precursor to entrance, is now an increasingly dominant mode of activity, substituting for the deep and tender feeling of coitus.

The use of anatomical parts not meant for sexual activity as a substitute for deep genital pleasure is another example of abuse. Sex that demands actual submission is violence. And to whip oneself, figuratively, into a frenzy of sexuality is as violent as if it were literal.

The most subtle acts of sexual violence are those that do not allow us to know what gendered sexuality is. Nothing has been more devastating than the medical and social-reform approaches to what sexuality should be. A well-known sex authority, for example, states that the arousal of the penis can come from any source, since it doesn't really know or care what arouses or satisfies it. Well, for the survival of the human species, the penis had better know what arouses it and where it should go.

It is often said that sex is like a thirst to be satisfied or an appetite to be slaked. Divorced from the act of bonding and the forming of relationships, sexual encounters have become "you do your thing and I will do mine, and off we go on independent ways." This is an act against personal integrity and one of violence and separation. If it is to maintain survival, the sexual act needs to be one of tenderness, caring, and understanding.

If we continue to deny our tenderness and longing, if we deny the fragility of loving, bonding, and child making, and if we insist on promoting a sexuality divorced from the evolution of these natural values, we will do more than reap violence. We must restore the primacy of bonding, and pass on to our young the truths of heterosexual relationship. From these deep satisfactions develop a life that is worth bringing children into, that they too may find their way to satisfaction and preserve the evolution of life without violence.

6 / Gender and Generation

IN THE earliest days of human embryological life, maleness and femaleness are set in place by hormones and chromosomes; these biological determinants baptize us as men or women and give us the deepest knowledge of the roles we are to play in the drama of evolution. The anatomical, hormonal, and emotional foundation that establishes individuality and differentiation is directly responsible for the roles we develop in the growth of the family and the emergence of the person.

Maleness and femaleness start out being essentially different in the quality of internal chemistry and in the geometry of anatomy. There is a hormonal disposition one way or the other; the waters are different, the quality of the living plasma is different. This leads to morphological and psychological differences. Early on, essential structures develop a different internal space. Within fifty days of conception, the differentiation between the male and the female body has been established. The basic hormonal disposition in the chromosomal patterns, XX–XY, results in a testosterone or estrogen predominance. Embryological, biochemical, and behavioral studies indicate that this predominance of male or female hormones is directly responsible for the development of testes or ovaries. This hormonal permeation interacting with the testes or ovaries has a tremendous impact upon the shape of the body and psyche. This interaction is directly responsible for the development of tissues and organs, including the central nervous system and the brain, into specifically male and female forms—developing a deeper pelvis or a narrower one, different muscle and fat patterns, and different qualities of brain tissue.

The sensations and feelings that grow out of these different internal spaces and forms provide another base for gender identity. The information of the uterus is different from the information coming from the penis or testes. And as reported in *Science* magazine's special issue on sexual dimorphism, even brain tissue develops specifically as male or female, giving rise to different perceptions and predispositions. There is, then, an embryologically based hormonal and anatomical thinking awaiting sociological experience. The information patterns from hormonal life and organ sensation give rise to behavior that, when met with parental caring and societal traditions, forms our emotional and psychological history.

Our hormonal tides lay down the first level of gender; then come the anatomical layers of tubes and muscle that give a second level, followed by sociological and personal history. These experiences are remembered deep in our tissues, giving rise to the holograms of our subjective psyches; and they help establish our identity, prepersonally, postpersonally, and personally. One is innately aware of this orientation.

Hormonal floods of testosterone or estrogen organize us toward male and female behavior: the erection of the penis, the release of the scent of estrus from the female, the bringing back of the pelvis to open the vaginal and uterine tubes. These predispositions have begun during the early weeks of life embryologically. Hormonal releases of androgen and estrogen give a feeling, a behavioral thrust to gender. Blood carries the secretions that give the generative organs their specific tubal motility, sending the sensations that state "I am a male" or "I am a female." These liquid floods are the flushes and waves of desire. This blood arousal, this cellular passion galvanizes gender. The fluids of the ductless glands are carried to all the organs where identity is based. To be more sexual does not mean being a performer; rather, it involves a powerful inward responsiveness of the prepersonal self—glands, brain, tubes, and hollows. These are the images and actions that organize gender.

Nature is not always right, and sometimes there is confusion. If body fluids lack sufficient hormones or the tissues of the testes, ovaries, and central nervous system do not interact with the correct sensitivity, the tissues may not galvanize as strongly male or female. The genitalia may be poorly formed, and the person may feel confused in his or her sexual orientation. The psyche may be in conflict with sensations from the genitalia and out of tune with society's demands.

Tubes and hollow spaces also have a good deal to do with how we perceive our gender. Male genitalia are external and extend outward, and the female's are internal and curve inward. In males, specific perceptions and behavior arise from spherical and tubal forms. The hollow spaces of the vagina and uterus generate feelings different to those produced by the pulsating tubes of the penis. One gives rise to a filled throbbing assertion, the other to a milking, filling feeling. The male feels the imperative to thrust, to expel, to fill; the woman feels the imperative to reach and to be filled.

The uterus is a vault, a hollow in which something happens that does not happen in the man — the generation of a life and its growth. That spaciousness, that hollowness is, in fact, a major determinant of femaleness; the space and feeling that grows out of it are dominant. Taking in, wanting to hold, to encase, to surround are dominant female feelings.

The movement of tubes assertively filling and emptying is the basic language of the inside of the body, transmitting experience directly. This geometry and the accompanying sensations are the tattoo of our maleness and femaleness. The full course of this language is an inherent knowledge accessible to us through our feelings. There is a gnawing dissatisfaction when the patterns of it are not lived. We know from the perceptions and behavior of our gender that it is the responsibility of the male to guarantee the generation of his seed and the transmission of it, and the responsibility of the female to guarantee the transmission of her eggs and the seeding of them. Of course, an individual may choose not to act on these directives, or to live them symbolically, but nevertheless they are the primal attitudes to take towards one's own gender and the surest means to maintain contact with one's sexuality.

Hormonal and morphological gender is confirmed by family and society. Nobody thinks a male or a female child is its opposite. We look at the genitalia and we understand that, in the course of time, this child will be a man or woman. Society demands certain kinds of behavior from children, treating them in a specific way within the family and within society at large, depending on whether they are male or female, and partially conditioning the manner in which individual biology will function. This societal conditioning cannot, however, be confused with the real hormonal, anatomical, and chromosomal bases on which sexual differences are based. If an individual's feeling of sexual identity grows out of societal role conditioning, that person may not have a feeling within the tissue of what his or her own maleness or femaleness is; sexuality becomes merely a remembrance of performance. The real strength of internal satisfaction comes from the intensity of hormones and tissue motility, which society either strengthens or weakens. No matter how one attempts to live out one's opposite (for example, a man who wants to be a woman), one's emotional intensity will never have the strength that comes from the development of what is given. If there is a dislike of one's gender, there may be pleasure in living out the opposite, and even a certain relief from conflict. But this assumed maleness or femaleness will lack the power poets have spoken of for millennia.

The true vitality of sexuality is dependent upon the quality of tone of the internal organs, and not upon the images we manufacture for ourselves. You can look sexy to the outside world, swing your pelvis, make a display of sexuality, and still be bereft of any internal sureness of gender. You can dress like a macho male, and the world will react to that image, but inside you may not feel it. The dress and the display are an attempt to generate a feeling within. It generally fails by leading one in the pursuit of images to satisfy, rather than feelings of satisfaction. This stimulant is unrelenting, and masks itself as feeling, often resulting in depression.

I have seen many people live overactive sexual lives, who, at the same time, complained of a lack of satisfaction and commitment. For them, sexuality offered the rewards of variety, but remained basically unsatisfying. Something was just not there. This complaint diminishes rapidly when tissue tone is improved and the quality of feeling that is engendered becomes the basis for contact, first with themselves, and then with another person.

The feeling of gender is dependent upon the unconscious or conscious perception of inner organs. The sensations of gender depend upon registering in the brain and psyche what is going on inside. Sexual identity is based upon the experiences of these sensations coming from the cells. The information of these sensations tattoos itself on the brain and makes a direct statement about one's gender. The essential point is that basic dysfunctions grow out of a misunderstanding or a misperception of one's own biological messages. Dysfunction is in the messages that emanate deep from one's own tissue. There is a relationship between the shape of the tissue and the programs in the brain. This means that there is a connection between what they were meant to do and what they are doing. The sexual organs grow from sexual cells, are placed in a functional position, and have a connection with the brain's programming. They represent a realm of experience that has been genetically transmitted.

Maleness and femaleness are the basic feelings and sensations that arise from inside the body and the genitalia. These feelings express gender, the urge of nature, and the urge of culture. This is an essential truth.

These simple facts of biological and emotional existence are under attack in the public arena. The media and the industry of pornography portray men and women in either an exaggerated or in an idealized fashion. The academic view of sexuality has become contaminated by the notion of neuter, leading to claims that the penis does not know the difference between self-stimulation and vaginal excitation, thus relegating the regular event that humans make babies either to chance or to sophisticated cortical knowledge. In the name of "science," sex research and education expose us to statements that are distorted when compared with the actual facts of existence. Does the penis not know the difference between the vagina and the anus or the oral cavity? Is it only social knowledge that conditions a woman to position herself for better contact between the penis and the vagina?

Another current view is that we are androgynous and bisexual. Here is a truth that has deep meaning on embryological, chemical, and symbolic levels. It has, however, been misinterpreted to the point where we believe that men can be women and women can be men, often resorting to surgical or chemical alterations. Levels of reality have become confused. In our attempts to create an egalitarian society, we have politicized and distorted gender. We live in a political climate that seeks to obliterate sexual differences, denouncing the concept of anatomy as destiny. By legislative fiat, society seeks to abandon maleness and femaleness, dismissing truths about differences and tensions known for ten thousand years of recorded history. This brings about an intellectual conception of equality, divorced from roots in experience or anatomy.

In our culture today, sexual identity is further compromised through the notion of "person." If I am a "person," I don't have to worry about my femaleness or maleness. I am a universal creature, for whom the values of being a person are more important than the values of being a *gendered* person. By denying the gender established by biochemical and anatomical states, sex research and education have exacerbated still further the contrast between society and the raw feelings of our real existence, all in the name of doing exactly the opposite. To streamline and make more efficient the transmission of sexual knowledge, society chooses to smooth out differences. But this does not ensure a greater understanding of what men and women are. The contrary is true. When there are no differences, no tensions between the sexes, vast holes of dissatisfaction and unmet longings emerge — a plague of emptiness that has us begging desperately for more of society's artificial stimuli to patch with some makeshift neural response what has become spent and undefined, lest we perish from lack of arousal.

Maleness and femaleness are a pattern of arousal that have endured since the beginning of human history. Gender seeks to again and again establish the conditions, the roles, and the behavior that guarantee the continuity of human life. From the well of gender comes the emotional passions for others and for life itself.

7 / Freedom and Destiny in Roles

SEXUAL roles are an innate part of life. On the prepersonal level, the hormonal and anatomical, they are established at conception. On the day of birth, "It's a boy! It's a girl!" announces the beginnings of social sexual identity. We look at the infant's genitalia and understand that, in the course of time, here will be a man or a woman. Society now starts to prepare the child for the expected sex roles.

This foundation — anatomical, hormonal, social — establishes how we act sexually, and will lead us toward the roles that provide satisfaction and sureness. Roles are the expression of hormonal and anatomical urges and the behavior whereby we create the social and personal patterns of our lives. Since gender is born in the prepersonal realm, the basic roles of male and female are given. Maturation and individuation, a combination of the given and the learned, is a development that occurs over time. This development of roles connects us to the prepersonal, initiates us into the social world, and gives us the opportunity to form a personal identity with individuality and freedom.

Roles are patterns of somatic organization that are purposeful behavior. Emotions and the urges of sexual hormones are complex behavior patterns and are the calls for action. Roles are the individual way we use muscle and brain together to create behavior. Our insides urge us to action, while society asks us to use ourselves to funnel energies and carry out tasks. Through the use of brain and muscle in concert, we learn the roles necessary for integrating the expectations of society with our own complex behavior patterns. This alchemical process, taking place over time, results in the finely integrated psychological, emotional, and muscular coordination that we call roles.

Roles support the development of feeling, of long-term bonding, and the development of family and community. They are the container for the deepening and the expression of sexual drives and emotional and sexual satisfactions. They also help establish order, perpetuate tradition, and provide security. Roles are regulators of social function, and they definitely are vital for the sexual rituals of reproduction and the development of love.

In the distant past, sex roles had to do simply with the behavior assigned by the estrogen-testosterone ritual. In early man, as throughout the animal kingdom, the female estrous cycle released the chemical signals that organized the whole reproductive act, establishing the given roles of penetrator and receptor. For whatever reason, the estrous cycle in human females became weakened, making possible year-round sexuality. This weakening of the estrous process, according to one author, J. Barnard, is what original sin is all about — approaching the woman out of her reproductive time.

It is highly significant that with the weakening of the hormonal ritual came the expansion of roles. Sexuality then became available for pleasure and connection, not just for conception. When the relationship of coitus to hormonal signals is disturbed, the set behavior and predictability of mating is lost. Instability and unsureness result. Here is the beginning of confusion between sex roles and gender. When roles are connected to hormonal and anatomical experience, there is little confusion on our part or on that of society about how we should behave. This elemental connection to gender — to the experience of hollows and liquids, the tides of reception and rushes of penetration — is a source of confidence and satisfaction. When feeling and action are integrated, we are nourished.

The importance of roles is that they are conduits and passageways for the parts that nature intends us to live. Most fundamentally, they constitute the behavior by which others recognize us in the game of reproduction. Gender creates the roles of replication. Without roles, there is no heterosexuality and no reproduction. The basic drama of male and female is the urge to penetrate and to receive, to fill and to empty. These feelings are the very basis of adult sexual encounters. Roles give us specific recognition from the opposite sex and connect us with the male world or the female world, endowing each with its own individual sexual identity.

Sexual roles are a continuum of forming. Powerful hormonal urges and anatomical development lead from infancy and childhood through adolescence into the world of adults. Somatic stimuli are the catalysts to developing the connections between prepersonal life and more personal and societal realms. The opportunity to mature in an individuated way requires the long development period of humans. In this relatively long formative time, there is the possibility to individuate the given and to mature inherent feelings and urges.

It is possible, of course, to adopt roles that imitate behavior. Many young people act as if they were older. Children, by observing the adults around them, in film, and on television, begin to practice sophisticated sex roles. They act "as if" without the physical, emotional, or psychological maturity to live out their actions. Adult sexual roles are, however, different from children's sexual posturing. Adult maturity is the ability to engage in emotional and instinctual behavior with high degrees of personal intimacy. Adult roles demand mutuality and a recognition of each person's patterns of assertion and pleasure.

People may also form roles that are vague in relation to one's own gender and that of the other. Frequently the role of adult is adopted to express an equality that has social, but not emotional, validity. There are big boys and big girls wanting to be treated as men and women, but not yet able to grasp the difference between the roles that are imitated and the realities that are generated by experience.

And there are those who deny their gender for economic, political, philosophical, or sexual reasons. Roles may be reversed, men acting as if they were women and women acting like men. Some people try to behave as neuters, calling themselves ascetics, androgynes, or simply "persons." These attempts to overcome anatomical destiny can be rewarding, but are often emotionally unsatisfying. In actuality, there is no neuter gender except through biological error or alteration. No matter what roles are assumed, body form identifies one person to another. The outward expression of gender can be changed to avoid the consequences of reproduction. One may seek protective roles such as those of philosopher, priest, nun, substitute mother, or spiritual leader to a group or country, but it is not possible to escape the destiny of gender totally.

From roles come a multiplicity of possibilities for individual achievement and personal freedom, for family bonding and shared intimacy, or for the misuse of self and even abuse of others. These choices become ours. Choice and freedom lie in either denying destiny or in evolving the possibilities of the male and female roles inherent in gender.

It is within the family that the quality of caring and emotional responsiveness most influences the ability to develop biologically rooted adult roles. The long tradition of reproductive behavior has established an ethic that gave birth to the family and the roles of mother, father, daughter, son, brother, sister, grandparents, aunts, uncles, and family-related friendships. It has also established rituals that are a clear rehearsal for adulthood. These familial roles establish clear performance expectations. They are also the ways we seek emotional bonding, connection, and extended caring. These caring roles bring about an enrichment of our gender, expanding the notion of mothering and fathering. Even though the roles we have today are becoming broader as we recognize the overlapping areas of competence between men and women, the models of sexual growth I have spelled out are not invalidated. Who is the breadwinner and who washes the dishes or bathes the children is not important. What is important is the dynamic of two different individuals with different innate functions that encourage emotional, biological, and personal roles fostering an enduring and loving coexistence. The differences of gender and how they form a personal style of male and female that determines the growth of the individual are the decisive point.

When roles are overbalanced, with too much emphasis on society or instinct, we are cut off from the full spectrum of life; we are left with a diminished or extinguished personal life. Living out instinctual urges cathartically results in poor role behavior in the social milieu. If we take on nothing more than the images of society, we become creatures of the pictures that are supplied to us, living only in our minds, not in our feelings. One can say, then, that the roles available to us are either the innate programmed imperatives of the prepersonal realm, the postpersonal roles imposed by society, or our personal adaptation somewhere in between. Today, more than ever before, we have increasing opportunity to develop our personal roles — we may be more libertarian, much more individualistic — but it is important to remember that our personal roles are deeply rooted in the prepersonal world and are very fragile. To protect and nourish our personal roles, we must know and respect their foundation. If we do not, prepersonal imperatives or postpersonal authority will take over and dominate. The roles we live today are multiple and diverse, but I do believe that the affirmation of heterosexual roles offers the promise of the richest expansion.

8 / The Contraceptive Ethic

MAN has sought to control his destiny since the dawn of his cortical awakening. With the understanding of the function of sperm and pregnancy and the discovery of the female ova, the control of human procreation took a leap forward. With the development of modern contraceptives and the safety of abortion, personal lives began to blossom. At the same time, the congruence of biological reality and human ethics began to change significantly. Religious, political, and social traditions had hitherto existed primarily as support for reproduction, the family, and the rearing of the young. These pervasive forces of the reproductive ethic are being challenged by a contraceptive minority and the growth of personal freedom.

There is now a clear contraceptive choice, taken by those who no longer wish to reproduce, those who delay their reproduction time, and those who want nothing to do with reproduction, but who still want a bonding relationship with the opposite sex. In the past eighty years, we have seen the emergence of a new set of rules for people, a changing of tradition, a redefining of sexual roles and destinies. Many names have been given to the phenomenon, but, to my knowledge, it has not been seen as the emergence of a third sex, the contracepted person. In support of this individual, there has also emerged a new, and now dominant, ethic — the ethic of contraception. It is recognizable in the deepening of the values of long-term education, and in the time available to devote to extended projects and to nourish them as one would nourish children. It is recognizable in the long-term investment we make in our offspring and the limited number of them. This is a key. Survival by numbers alone has been replaced with survival by the well-trained and specialized few. This contraceptive dimension is an outgrowth of the development of the personal realm that seeks to be free from the tyranny of the pre- and postpersonal dogmas.

For most of our population, contraception has been successful in allowing choices beyond the two extremes of unrestrained reproduction or sexual abstinence. The contraceptive choice represents the continuity of the personal caring and development experienced in our families and our institutions. Indeed, this ethic supports the pursuit of some of mankind's highest freedoms. Yet it is this very pursuit, in the extreme, that distorts the nature of freedom and perverts the rules of nature. Sexuality based on the powerful urges for reproduction and emotional bonding becomes sex for personal gratification with no connection to the past or future.

History is filled with nonreproductive men and women. In the tradition of the monastic elite, the goal was to transcend anatomy—to deny biological heritage and transform sexual desire and familial obligation into spiritual enlightenment. Freedom from biological imperatives was represented in platonic love, in the ancient love of men for men, and in the philosophical and historical attempt to mute the instinctual prepersonal life in the interests of a private, personal world. Nonreproduction, then, represented the fulfillment of personal goals. Efforts to free oneself from the rules and bonds of the prepersonal and postpersonal realms were conducted either by imitating a nonreproductive physical relationship or by diverting sexual energies into other roles, such as the celibate priest, who could act as a nourishing father. The ordained religious became spiritual mothers and fathers.

The cultivation of the personal world was the gift of the intelligentsia and the visionaries, the elite class of any given society. It was the possession of those who understood that there were initiations into a secret world, and that the bond between mother and child was not simply to safeguard the latter, but included the transmission of experience and wisdom. The ascetics used parenting models to conceive ideas, and to grow them. Their reproductive urge was sublimated in the service of the spirit to evolve a family of kindred seekers, a brotherhood. Unfortunately, in the extreme, these disciplines generated a hatred of the flesh and a fear of the opposite sex.

Now modern contraception has opened the door to the widespread establishment of the personal world as a domain in and of itself, and a possibility for the many. The personal world that previously was based upon great sacrifice has now become an ordinary event. Contraception makes the personal world available to all. We can still engage in sex and stay free of the reproductive consequences, and even accept assigned sexual roles and escape nature's will. We can bond or couple and not reproduce, and thereby build lives that use sex for pleasure and intimacy alone. The opportunity to take on, and live out, roles not connected to one's anatomy is an enormous step forward in the realm of freedom.

Nearly all of us, at one time or another, live a contracepted life. In delaying family, there is a valuable and rich opportunity to enjoy the broad spectrum of personal fulfillment. Contraception is a valid attempt to regulate and to enhance one's life. But, in pursuing freedom from the imperative of reproduction, there is a risk of creating a personal life in which gender is blurred.

Gender is the ingredient that determines the relationship between the sexes, and it is being challenged by today's concept of the "person." The person is supposed to be free of maleness or femaleness, a sort of ideal ego state, lacking biological and emotional gender. This notion of the person has entered the political, legal, and judicial areas, where equality is meant to overcome discrimination according to gender. The idea of equal opportunity within our laws and institutions has been extended, and has come to be interpreted to mean that males and females are equal biological and emotional beings. We have created a mythological, nonsexed person with no base in biological reality, derived only from political, legal, and sexual fantasy. Contraception further weakens roles based on gender and on the primacy of biology and makes possible this third sex, the non-reproductive person playing nonreproductive roles.

It is from these concepts and attitudes that our society presently receives definitions of what gender is, and, more specifically, what it should not be and what families should or should not be. This fiddling around with sex roles has implications that have not been clearly articulated.

The contraceptive ethic postulates an androgynous world and then creates institutions that back it up. Many of the distortions today—in schools, courts, unions, government regulations—stem from non-gendered ideals. Schools now wish to instruct children in sexual behavior before their bodies and emotions are ready, giving them the permission and the right to adult behavior. On a more subtle level, the contraceptive ethic has made us more tolerant of child pornography and violent and overtly sexual films and television; it has also contributed to the devaluation of child rearing and breastfeeding, and to the substitution for mothers of someone called a "primary care person."

The contraceptive ethic states clearly that the growth and gratification of the personal self is the most important value and one that the institutions should now reflect. The inherent statement is that we must protect the now and not the future. This ethic makes the collective vision of the reproductive ethic obsolete, because it discourages investment in the future. The contraceptive ethic must denigrate the past, since it seeks to overcome it. It must see the future in terms of its own view, since it is not committed to reproductive continuity unless the goal — the longing for children — is kept alive.

The contraceptive ethic has become a strong voice in the United States and seeks to impose its values on the total population the way the reproductive ethic has done in all the rest of the world. The lines of battle are seen in the abortion and anti-abortion fights. There are those people who say that the body is their private property and their choices are theirs alone, and those who say that the body belongs to God and society. These issues are a reflection of the emergence of the contracepted person who is seeking to have his rights heard.

The contraceptive choice is more dominant now because more people in the United States are not part of the reproductive realm either by reason of age, choice, or anatomical difficulties. One of the main messages they send is that they do not wish to be discriminated against if they do not marry or if they do not have children. And, of course, these sexual expressions and demands are valid. Unfortunately, many of the attitudes that seek to make the contraceptive ethic accepted and dominant at the same time act to deflate the reproductive base of nature and to place reproduction, biological roles, and gender in the political arena.

The danger in delaying reproductive urges and in promoting contraception divorced from the fullness of human relationships and evolution is that we run the risk of generating an ethic in which sexuality becomes disembodied. What was a vision born of freedom from instinct becomes the vehicle for sex as an activity to be exploited.

Sex is the container for our deepest intimacies and most intense human connections; yet, when it is used as an isolated excitatory catharsis or momentary erotic stimulation, psyches become unbounded and debased images of sexuality flood the human world. In the indiscriminate living out of sexual impulses, the opportunity to act from the messages of our gender and from the depth of emotional satisfaction is lost. Sex becomes an idealized activity exploited by external stimulation. We see this in the obvious over-stimulation produced and demanded by our culture, in the uses of sex far removed from enriching personal maturation or forming enduring relationships. Sex has become a thing in itself and there is a constant seeking for variety, new techniques for arousal, and the substitution of fantasy for contact. Relationship is unimportant, a future is unimportant. Sex is done for sex itself. This is not freedom, but a misdirected use and outcome of contraception.

The use of fantasy in the pursuit of sexual adventure is not free of consequences. In the acting out of a sexuality unrelated to gender and its deepest biological message, a type of impersonality emerges. When men and women have little or no connection to their biological roots and are unable to use the innate perceptions available to them from their gender, they can only act from the undifferentiated instinctual patterns of the prepersonal world or in imitation of societal images. The personal freedom to mediate these two worlds is lost, and the highest purpose of contraception is defeated.

There are more subtle and pervasive influences that undermine the nature of our humanness, all in the name of freedom and enlightenment. One is the attitude promoted by the Population Zero people that having children or multiple children is anti-survival. Women are discouraged from becoming mothers when career achievement and personal gratifications are valued above the creation of a family and the nurturing of human life. Women who stay at home to raise children are demeaned, and even the temporary sacrifice of personal freedom required to raise small children is considered an unnecessary burden. The current ideal female form is the opposite of the fullness of a pregnant or lactating woman, the fertility figure of old. Today's fashion demands thin bodies and ones that look perpetually young. Clothing styles accurately reflect the unisex pubescent ideal.

Male and female relationships are further diminished in the laboratory as genetic engineering and techniques for nonsexual reproduction and in vitro fertilization develop. And I have already discussed the attempts to replace male and female with a neuter gender, the "person," on the legal and political levels of society. The truth of specialized behavior and roles based in the given of our reproductive natures and rooted in gender cannot be ignored without serious consequences.

I have made strong statements that males and females have different experiences and perceptions. And I similarly believe that people who have children have a different experience of sexuality from those who do not have children or who delay family making. Make no mistake, these can be valid and good choices, but the two groups have different perceptions and make different choices. Today the perceptions and interests representing the nonreproducing segment are dominant and are thrust upon the rest of society the way the values of the reproducers used to be. I support those who choose not to have children that are not wanted or cannot be raised well; however, my concern is that there are few people making statements in support of heterosexuality and enduring family relationships, a view that needs strong affirmation in our times.

What really concerns me is the blatant and heedless interference in the human sexual process and the way it is reflected in how we teach our children. Public educators and policy makers subscribe to a program that teaches anatomy and physiology and instructs in sex play, while leaving out the powerful forces of human interaction. Nothing is said about the ability to withhold one's self, or how to resist peer pressure; or how struggling with a force larger than yourself is an impetus to maturity. Public instruction says that contraception makes us all equal, youngsters as well as adults, regardless of whether one is emotionally prepared for sexual activity. We encourage long-term dependency in our children and promote their sexual rights and protection, but we do not include emotional maturity or rights. We are more interested in cognitive maturity, and end up dismissing hundreds of years of human experience about sex bonding and lifestyle.

Now we are faced with children wanting their sexual rights. Society feels they should have access to contraceptive materials and be allowed to experiment sexually. This will happen, does happen; children and young people will not be stopped. But there seems to be a Machiavellian intent to encourage childhood sex that is fostered by adults and unrelated to the natural desires of children. This, of course, is crazy. There should be strong family and social education as to the deeper possibilities of sex, love, and the forming of emotional bonds. The practice of public education requires a commitment to personal and societal humanity. It does not require the pushing of a viewpoint for the sake of personal pleasure or simply to be free of disease and pregnancy.

The promise of contraception—to delay childbearing or to prevent it for all sorts of personal and societal reasons—is a tremendous boon. It escalates the power of personal maturity and growth. It helps regulate survival and continuity in times of great stress. It contributes greatly to the store of human experience and knowledge and offers a true hope for the realization of humanness. Man reveals himself through continuing intimacy, and contraception makes this possible. But the power of these options cannot be allowed to savage the heterosexual imperative, which is, after all, the coexistence of two different world views. Nature expresses unity in diversity. Diversity prospers not as competition but as cooperation.

Our institutions should seek to protect our children and a gendered human species. The use of contraception need not in the least diminish the profound and ancient origins of sexual destiny, nor the importance of the prepersonal domain in forming that destiny and an orientation toward life. Heterosexuality is a given that has the chance to develop through all the realms of existence. To know this, to live this, is a human need. Heterosexuality is our anchor to the source of life. It is reality, and without a doubt links us to a future.

9 / Family-Making

IN ALL of human history, the primary connection between men and women has been the urge to mate. Gender is what has enabled people to recognize one another in order to carry out their roles in this drama. Reproduction has always been the goal, whether it was known or not.

One of the important functions of sex is to create bonds and connections. For gamete cells to join requires only short-term bonding; ejaculation requires a few seconds to do its work of fertilization. Why, then, does a man need to be around afterwards? In the lower animal world, the male usually does not remain with his mate after ejaculation. Ascending the scale of evolution into the realm of warm-blooded animals, however, sex takes on other functions. Through the development of parental caring, it becomes the vehicle for deep bonds and emotional connections. Sexuality is like a placenta; it joins and nourishes the growth of the self and others, and generates blood rituals in which people exchange emotional and psychological nourishment, enter each other, and create a field of feeling. We establish pathways or tunnels to pass back and forth the ingredients of growth and nourishment. This bonding activity is part and parcel of human activity; it is family-making.

The history of warm-bloodedness and heat regulation is also the history of maternal caring. With maternal caring, the heat of the womb is maintained from the outside. The closeness of the parent's body permits the infant's heat regulation to be more constant. This makes growth and learning more stable. Parents and families are like wombs, sustaining warmth, allowing caring to develop into love. Human sexuality is the bringer of warmth.

The function of family is to act as an incubator, to insure heat via emotional and nutritional interaction that permits tissue and personality growth. The family is a structure that provides stable, continuous warmth through physical and emotional contact, and this in turn encourages the development of personal behavior. The development of warm-blooded behavior—of personal caring—brings into being an individual, a personal existence rather than a collective one.

This familial bonding has introduced into society a set of experiences that has had the effect of reorganizing sexual experience, making it a multi-leveled event. One of the important events of human history has been the evolution of the family and the powerful galvanizing force of reproductive couples. With the development of the family began the traditions which made sexuality a continuum, which extended it from impersonal connections to societal forms and to the concept of a childhood that is personal and intimate.

The roles that accompanied these traditions became the norm. The father as breadwinner, the mother as sacrificer; paternal love and maternal love; the primacy of the eldest son—all these notions came into existence and were important in developing personal identities.

The family, this complex and dominant shaper of individuals and society, has always had its problems and challenges. The dichotomy between long-term relationships and sexual adventure has existed in the family since its beginnings. Many conflicts arose between sex and caring; incest and fidelity became a serious social concern. This conflict has gained in intensity because of effective contraception, the broadening of society's sexual codes, and frantic attempts to reconnect with something real. Sexual diversity has a strong voice in nature, one that cannot be easily dismissed. At the same time, heterosexuality and the family create stability and intimacy through exclusivity. Diversity and exclusivity are the essential parameters of growth. Each person must come to terms with his own emotional truth.

Now, new challenges face couples and families. Until quite recently, the family perpetuated itself through such ideas and functions as the right to rule, the orderly transference of power, satisfaction of economic needs, and the generation of work units, of which children were an important part.

For many reasons, these historical family roles are breaking down; certainly the increasing emphasis on individuality, freedom, and personal satisfaction contributes to the fading away of traditional family systems. Most men and women today form emotional bonds based on love and choice rather than upon reproduction and economics. And there are the added factors of long-term education, extended periods of dependency, increased mobility, economic opportunity, and freedom from sexual consequences through abortion and contraception. People no longer marry primarily to have children, either for the joy of raising them or to make an economic unit. Now couples demand more from each other. They want intimacy, sexual fulfillment, individuality, social access, economic freedom, companionship, and careers as well as shared child rearing roles. Psychological compatibility is as important as sexual compatibility. With this concentration of demands, heterosexual roles begin to collapse, and powerful stresses enter the family structure.

This is a transitional time for family structure, and we have yet to see the maturation of the possibilities. What we do see now is experimentation and confusion in family-making. World War II did much to hasten change in American families, and in the last generation, freedom and opportunity have allowed a new societal permissiveness, unheard of before the War. Couples can live together openly without marriage; unmarried women can have children without public censure; the gay rights movement has made possible more open homosexual coupling; contraception has made recreational and casual sex an everyday opportunity.

Out of these choices, a new kind of bonding emerges, one that rivals the traditional family. Two people come together for longer or shorter periods of time to satisfy their personal needs for physical, sexual, and emotional contact. The strength of their connection is based on the recognition of the need for intimacy and sexual pleasure without having to choose child rearing.

This new dimension of living, contracepted living, has generated confusion about the function of sexuality as well as what the family is, what gender is, and what sexual roles are. Without doubt, we are witnessing the disintegration of the household and, as a consequence, the isolation of sexuality. Wendell Berry, an eloquent commentator on the human condition, puts it this way, in *The Unsettling of America:*

The division of sexual energy from the functions of household and community that it ought both to empower and to grace is analogous to that other modern division between hunger and the earth. When it is no longer allied by proximity and analogy to the nurturing disciplines that bound the household to the cycles of fertility and the seasons, life and death, then sexual love loses its symbolic or ritualistic force, its deepest solemnity and its highest joy. It loses its sense of consequence and responsibility. It becomes "autonomous," to be valued only for its own sake, therefore frivolous, therefore destructive — even of itself. Those who speak of sex as "recreation," thinking to claim for it "a new place," only acknowledge its displacement from Creation.

What, then, is the future of sexuality, of the family? What sort of human units will emerge that can weather the psychological images and the lure of physical freedom? No one can know for sure, but I am certain that bonding and intimacy are urgent human needs, needs that are deep within the genes and tissues. The urge to form family is the companion of reproductive instincts. The repression or weakening of this urge has the same effect on human happiness and emotional and bodily sanity as the distortion of the sexual impulse. We are not meant to be alone, and the urges for mating and family-making are very present, though often hidden under a blanket of social precepts.

One new family form, already in evidence, is characterized by a delayed reproductive life. Since procreative urges are easily amended in these contra-cepted times, many women are conceiving their first children much later than did their mothers a generation ago. The 1980 census shows that the birthrates of women over 35 have increased by 45 percent. Many children will have older, presumably more mature and experienced, parents. Another family form is a single, unmarried woman (and sometimes a man) with a child. Instead of coping with a love for an equal and an opposite, the parent has a child who becomes the adored one, the sole recipient of love and caring. In the extreme, these parent-child connections become part of Christopher Lasch's "culture of narcissism."

We are very fortunate to live in a time that allows so many individual choices and supports broader, more tolerant social notions. The reproductive imperative and the goals of family-making do not cancel out the personal choices of the homosexual, the ascetic, and the childless individual. But family-making remains a crucial function for a vital and evolving society and one our institutions need to affirm. Family life that supports psychological, emotional, and individual growth, while also providing intimacy and stability, is an ideal and a possibility rooted in the heterosexual connection and the emotional bonds it is capable of establishing. The human family is a somatic, emotional collective that functions to continually reproduce and form itself.

10 / In Defense of Heterosexuality

WHY does heterosexuality need to be so vigorously affirmed? Not to preserve the rituals of marriage and family, for these have separate traditions, but to affirm that bonding and commitment are at the very core of human existence. In my understanding, heterosexuality and the basic sexual reproductive roles are the way nature exhibits order. The basic urges toward bonding bring about an understanding of ourselves and nature and give meaning to our lives. I speak not of a conceptualized philosophy, but of a deep somatic and emotional base that gives rise to the proven perceptions that have resulted in the perpetuation of life, society, and individuals.

Humans have always had a deep and powerful intuitive sense of how life worked, and seeking knowledge about the nature of life has been the concern of all people at all times. To grapple with death, creation, nourishment, children — all have to do with an ethic of life. And it is no different today. In affirming our heterosexual heritage, we are perpetuating a view of the world.

Life is a formative process, ever transcending

styles of existence on the personal and societal levels, yet remaining remarkably constant in its organizing emotional form. The dance of opposing forces — male and female — engenders personal and societal destiny. In the coming together of sexual opposites, we have an ancient and timeless way to reproduce, grow, and maintain the body. This pattern of reproduction is the root pattern of biological existence, the basis of genetic and human knowledge.

Heterosexuality, then, is a statement of a basic law of nature. It is an expression of male and female modes of existence and of how polarization, specialization, and bonding bring about humanness.

Our inner organs give rise to patterns of arousal and motility and to the emotions that make us male or female. The natural differences are seen in the shape of human bodies: male bodies differ from females in their fat distribution, in their muscle size, in the shape of the pelvis, in the anatomy of their genitalia. We know maleness and femaleness in behavior specialization, like erection or lactation, and certainly we know it in the sexual act. In the copulatory movements, the specialty of our gender is further revealed. There is a difference between entering and being entered, the movement of penetration and the movement of taking in. There are different patterns of arousal for man and woman. Human survival rests upon our ability to have knowledge of existence different from another's existence, and for these poles of separateness to find a way to coexist. Heterosexuality is the language of the union of opposites in a pattern that serves reproduction and evolution, that is continuity, growth, intimacy, and separateness. It is thus a pattern for creation and a model for living, be it literal or symbolic.

The basic function of heterosexuality is to bring men and women together, to foster shared experience, to join chromosomal and genetic experience, to perpetuate life. It is the force that holds men and women together to create an environment for offspring to mature in. This interaction initiates the caring, contactful dialogues that help humans grow as gendered persons.

Heterosexuality is reproduction for survival. With the beginning of long-term bonding and the introduction of personal caring came the union of sex and tenderness and the evolution of a personal relationship. And that personal relationship develops into what we call love. This love then extends to members of our immediate family, to ourselves, and to other members of our planet. Heterosexuality is the evolution of love.

Our human institutions are in a state of destructuring and reforming. The fundamentals of individuation — gender, commitment, family, long-term caring — are being challenged. We seem to seek to deny the very basis of human uniqueness. We can, and do, transcend our personal and societal destinies; this is our history, our human heritage. We form and then reform personal and postpersonal existence, but I doubt if we can rearrange gender and its roles or deflect the bonding and parenting urges without negatively altering our future.

When a sexual ethic is formed separate from nature, distortion occurs. Not only the sexual function is disturbed, but a world view as well. The question then becomes, is there something sacred and instinctual that gives us an orientation? Heterosexuality, as I have described it, is not only mutual servicing or mutual delight. It is the enactment of the passion of union. It is the exchange of the cells of our immortality.

Heterosexuality sets the model for a social order. But today, partly because of the success of contraception, we think we can desert this truth. Contraception was meant to delay reproduction so that the realm of personhood and individuality could grow. I have said that concern for the growth of the individual as represented by the contraceptive ethic, by the non-reproductive life, has in its own right deepened private life. But the contraceptive ethic has also weakened the bonds of our biological history, and now tries to dominate sexual reality.

When people choose not to reproduce or to delay reproduction until they feel mature enough to have children, they may lose contact with the urgency of the basic desire for replication. There is then the danger of losing the feelings which form the connections that permit emotional bonding and its responses as guides for the evolution of ourselves and society. The lack of love, passion, and loyalty are a result of the domination of what I have called the contraceptive ethic and lifestyle.

Not so long ago, large families and extended familial relationships were the order of the day. Yet now we have moved away from the compelling need to make union and are taught to devalue the development of enduring relationships and the raising of families. This dominant theme of independence needs to come closer to the truth of interdependence. When sexuality takes on the layers of the shared experiences of familial life, it becomes the incubator of personal caring and nurturing. It brings to the foreground the emotional intensities that become part and parcel of lovemaking. Lovemaking is the sharing of personal experience and is meant to form emotional bonds that in turn encourage the transmission of experience to one's offspring—that is, to the future.

Heterosexual bonding is the way for most of us. It is an order that is flexible in humans, but this flexibility is also capable of misuse. Many people are trying to orient themselves through mistaken notions of freedom. We think we are sexually liberated today, but this is not at all the case. The forces of sexual hate are rampant in the form of degrading heterosexuality, in divorcing sex from children and love. With the sexualization of everything, we downgrade the notions of reproduction and growth of intimacy. When we make sexual delight most important, we confuse the nature of heterosexuality.

Human prepersonal, instinctual patterns set the ground and the tone on which one can build a personality and an individual life. There is, then, a natural order to which mankind is bound, not imprisoned. Only lower forms of life are locked into a program. Human sexuality is a continuum of nature—animal, human, and self. Unless we understand this, we are in danger of becoming lower animals only. Love is the mark of our humanness.

The development of humanity requires long-term parenting and the internalization of experience. The expression of human heterosexuality is seen in the face-to-face copulatory pattern, where the exchange of intimacy and feelings communicates the internal experience of the partners. This face-to-faceness, this learning of extended fondness through the sharing of experience is also present in the mother-child relationship. The human infant spends more time than any other creature looking at the face of its mother. Here is intimacy functioning as the evoker of response and long-term relationship.

Human sexuality is distinguished by the development of an inner life. Individuality and personhood grow from a biological basis that fires the imagination and creates the conditions of inner vision and perspective. Human sexuality is unique in uniting a biochemical chromosomal sexuality, a mammalian warm-blooded, caring sexuality of connection and companionship, and the human ability to personalize nature. The ability of our species to internalize and personalize through memory, imagery, and voluntary action creates the conditions for arousal of self and other. This inner eye of images, of past and future, creates situations that generate a personal world. This is the special condition that expands nature's rigid, biochemical, genetic reproductive rules, and gives meaning by permitting the establishment of societal and personal order.

Society has tried to encourage order by regulating the sex act and enforcing parenting. Yet in this attempt to help, society has imposed a use of our bodies that has been repressive, and represents a misuse of our sexuality and gender. So today we have tried to pry sexuality from the old traditions by returning to a picture of mindless sex. In this attempt to free ourselves, we have made the serious error of giving up the internal experience of sexuality. We know ourselves sexually by the shape of the inside and outside of our bodies, by our inner movements and urgings. We know we are human by our ability to have images, feelings that we can reflect upon, cherish, and reenact.

Our humanness is being eroded by instant history, in which one never gets a chance to reflect on an experience before another is shoved down one's throat, so that people become nothing more than instant moments; they never have a chance to allow their experience to deepen and grow. To learn to reorganize oneself out of one's past is very different from severing oneself from the past and jumping from one instant into the next.

Most people are not oriented to learn from their internal experience, their somatic history. Our institutions and the media have made public and political every biological act. There has been an attempt to abort the private, personal continuum of growth, to define freedom by making every act public, and to pressure people into the ethic of sexuality as non-reproductive and non-gendered. We are not encouraged to grow into our own sexual maturity. We are told what our sexual rights are, and then commanded to take them. How can that be? Our sexual rights are to copulate for reproduction, and our rights as a person are to use our sexuality to bring us satisfaction. But this growth—this learning—does not require that we be told what to do and how to do it.

The public domain has been extended deep into

our somas; slogans and pictures enter our brains and viscera. The private domain is being wiped out by the political and media pictures of what should be inside. Our lives are dominated by public pressure to behave in specific ways in all our acts, including working, copulating, and even dying. And with this intrusion has come the disruption of the basic feeling of our heterosexual heritage, the disruption of the fruits of caring, individuality, and loving that mark our humanness.

Heterosexuality is nature's design for the evolution of a personal dimension; to be under the imperative to reproduce brings the values of birth, creation, growth, and dying into the foreground of every human life. Heterosexuality is an ongoing drama not only of replication, but of birth and death, destiny and choice, determinism and freedom, cultural and personal values. This heterosexual reality unites carnality and spirit, desire and vision. Thus we know nature, self-nature, and human nature from our insides.

We can choose to make sex impersonal, to permit sexuality to exist simply as a mechanism for pleasure, and to return to a prepersonal world; or we can choose to see sexuality as an act of love, accompanied by the formation of emotional bonds and the evolution of our humanness through the life of relationship and the life of the family. The choice is between two world views—one which understands that the world is becoming more human, and one which asserts that the world always has been and always will be an impersonal globe in space.

Heterosexuality should not be confused with

marriage or with family in the traditional legal sense. It should be conceived as a gendered, anatomical, psychological, emotional process, whose continuity depends upon both separateness and closeness, a polar dynamic that makes connections of wholeness. Heterosexuality, then, is the process of union and the continuation of this union to the development of an intimate, multi-leveled, enduring relationship that has among its fruits child bearing, child rearing, and a commitment to the future of humanness.

Heterosexuality is the infrastructure of passion, of desire; the compelling feeling to bond, the core of the primitive mothering, caring, and paternal instincts. It has a great deal to teach us. Heterosexuality has an anatomy, a chemistry, a psychology, and a specific behavior, which I have described. I have shown how the biological thread of human anatomical history reveals the way human perception exposes its truth, both concretely and symbolically. Heterosexuality is a frame of reference to grow from, a place to create from, a place to learn from. As a way of existence, it has brought tremendous fruits — culture, art, science, and love — into being. It denies no other lifestyle, but without it no other human life may endure.

Heterosexuality needs to be affirmed as the heart of human life. I believe it is imperative that men and women recognize that the roots of civilization and culture are deep in the reproductive imperative. It has conceived, nurtured, and extended reproduction into intimacy and caring, into the noble truth of love and friendship. It has tried, and still tries, to make the biosphere a mantle of human caring.

Bibliography

Beach, F. A., ed., *Human Sexuality in Four Perspectives*, Johns Hopkins University Press, Baltimore, 1976.

Bennett, W. J., "Teaching the Young About Sex," *American Educator*, Winter 1980, Volume 4, Number 4.

Bernard, J., *The Sex Game*, Prentice Hall, Englewood Cliffs, New Jersey, 1968.

Berry, W., *The Unsettling of America*, Sierra Club Books, 1977.

Blechschmidt, E., *The Beginnings of Human Life*, Springer Verlag, New York, 1977.

Bonaparte, M., *Female Sexuality*, International Universities Press, New York, 1953.

Boss, M., *Meaning and Content of Sexual Perversion*, Grune & Stratton, New York, 1949.

Branden, N., *The Psychology of Romantic Love*, J. P. Tarcher, Inc., Los Angeles, 1980.

Bullough, V. L., *The Subordinate Sex*, Penguin Books, Baltimore, 1974.

Deutsch, H., *Neuroses and Character Types*, Hogarth Press, London, 1965.

Dinnerstein, D., *The Mermaid and the Minotaur*, Harper & Row, New York, 1976.

Duyckaerts, F., *The Sexual Bond*, Delacorte Press, New York, 1970.

Foucault, M., *The History of Sexuality*, Vintage Books, New York, 1980.

Hogan, R. and D. Schroeder, "The Joy of Sex for Children and Other Modern Fables," *Character*, August 1980, Volume 1, Number 10.

Hunt, M. M., *The Natural History of Love*, Alfred A. Knopf, New York, 1959.

Keleman, S., *The Human Ground: Sexuality, Self and Survival*, Center Press, Berkeley, California, 1975.

Keleman, S., *Your Body Speaks Its Mind*, Center Press, Berkeley, California, 1975.

Lasch, C., *Haven in a Heartless World*, Basic Books, Inc., New York, 1977.

Lederer, W. J. and Jackson, D., *Mirages of Marriage*, W. W. Norton, New York, 1968.

Lederer, W., *The Fear of Women*, Grune & Stratton, New York, 1968.

Lowen, A., *Love and Orgasm*, Signet Books, New York, 1963.

Lynn, D. B., *The Father: His Role in Child Development*, Wadsworth Publishing Co., Monterey, California, 1974.

Mahler, M. S. and Pine, F., and Bergman, A., *The Psychological Birth of the Human Infant*, Basic Books, New York, 1975.

Mantegazza, P., *Sexual Relations of Mankind*, Eugenics Publications, New York, 1935.

Masters, W. J. and V. E. Johnson, *Human Sexual Response*, Little, Brown, 1966.

May, R., *Sex and Fantasy*, W. W. Norton, New York, 1980.

Midghey, M., *Beasts and Man*, Cornell University Press, Ithaca, New York, 1978.

Money, J. and Ehrhardt, A., *Man and Woman, Boy and Girl*, Johns Hopkins University Press, Baltimore, 1972.

Money, J., *Sex Errors of the Body*, Johns Hopkins University Press, Baltimore, 1968.

Mott, F. J., *The Little History*, Mark Beech Publishers, Kent, United Kingdom, 1970.

Naftolin, F. and E. Butz, eds., "Sexual Dimorphism" *Science*, March 20, 1981, Volume 211, No. 4488.

Peck, M. S., *The Road Less Traveled*, Simon & Schuster, New York, 1978.

Reich, W., *The Function of the Orgasm*, Orgone Institute Press, New York, 1948.

Sexton, P., *The Feminized Male*, Random House, New York, 1969.

Symons, D., *The Evolution of Human Sexuality*, Oxford University Press, New York, 1979.

Szasz, T., *Sex by Prescription*, Anchor Press/Doubleday, Garden City, New York, 1980.

Tannahill, R., *Sex in History*, Stein & Day, New York, 1980.

von Urban, R., *Sex Perfection and Marital Happiness*, The Dial Press, New York, 1949.

Center For Energetic Studies

The Center for Energetic Studies in Berkeley, California, under the direction of Stanley Keleman seeks to structure a modern contemplative approach to self-knowing and living in which one's own subjective process gives birth to a set of values which then guides the whole of one's life. Today's values are increasingly divorced from our deepest processes, and bodily experience has been misunderstood and relegated to second place.

Somatic reality is an emotional reality that is much larger than innate genetic patterns of behavior. Emotional reality and biological ground are the same and cannot, in any way, be separated or distinguished. Biological ground also means gender, the male and female responses that are innate to human life, the sexual identity with which we are born. Somatic reality is at the very core of existence, the source of our deepest religious feelings and psychological perceptions.

Classes and programs at the Center offer a psycho-physical practicum that brings to use the basic ways a person learns. The key issue is *how* we use ourselves—learning the language of how viscera and brain use muscle to create behavior. These classes teach the essential somatic aspect of all roles and dramatize the possibilities of action to deepen the sense of connection to the many worlds in which all of us participate.

For further information, write to:
Center for Energetic Studies
2045 Francisco Street
Berkeley, California 94709

Available From Center Press

BOOKS
by Stanley Keleman

Somatic Reality	$ 7.95
Your Body Speaks Its Mind	7.95
Living Your Dying	5.95
Human Ground/Sexuality, Self and Survival	5.95
Todtmoos: A Book of Poems	2.00

by Tamara Greenberg and Anne Lief Barlin

Move and Be Moved	15.00

TAPES
Audio cassette tapes of Keleman workshops.

Trust versus Self reliance (includes written transcript)	12.95
Containment (includes written transcript)	12.95
On Touching and Exercise (90 Minute audio tape)	7.50
Somatic Process and Nature of the Soul (two 90 minute audio tapes)	15.00

MONOGRAPHS

Clinical Studies in Somatic Process: Movement and Motility; Somatic Process and Resistance; Possessiveness and Possessedness	3.50
Clinical Studies in Somatic Process: Somatic Initiation; Human Bodyhood; Toward a New Psychology	4.50

JOURNAL
Edited by Ian J. Grand.

Journal of Somatic Experience, published twice yearly	14.00/yr